T0208811

# POLYGAMY: IS IT A KILLER?

# POLYGAMY: IS IT A KILLER?

## The Voices of Ten American-Based Nigerian Women

*Christy 'Seyi Olorunfemi, PhD*

iUniverse®

**POLYGAMY: IS IT A KILLER?**
**THE VOICES OF TEN AMERICAN-BASED NIGERIAN WOMEN**

*Copyright © 2017 Christy 'Seyi Olorunfemi, PhD.*

*All rights reserved. No part of this book may be used or reproduced by any means, graphic, electronic, or mechanical, including photocopying, recording, taping or by any information storage retrieval system without the written permission of the author except in the case of brief quotations embodied in critical articles and reviews.*

*iUniverse books may be ordered through booksellers or by contacting:*

*iUniverse*
*1663 Liberty Drive*
*Bloomington, IN 47403*
*www.iuniverse.com*
*1-800-Authors (1-800-288-4677)*

*Because of the dynamic nature of the Internet, any web addresses or links contained in this book may have changed since publication and may no longer be valid. The views expressed in this work are solely those of the author and do not necessarily reflect the views of the publisher, and the publisher hereby disclaims any responsibility for them.*

*Any people depicted in stock imagery provided by Thinkstock are models, and such images are being used for illustrative purposes only.*
*Certain stock imagery © Thinkstock.*

*ISBN: 978-1-5320-1868-8 (sc)*
*ISBN: 978-1-5320-1867-1 (e)*

*Library of Congress Control Number: 2017905017*

*Print information available on the last page.*

*iUniverse rev. date: 04/27/2017*

*To my dear husband 'Segun and lovely children,*
*Ayobami, Ayodeji, and Ayokunle, for their*
*support and love during this process*

# ACKNOWLEDGMENTS

I give thanks to God for all of my accomplishments. I appreciate the support of my family and other people who have made this milestone possible through their prayers and words of encouragement.

# PREFACE

This book is about polygamy and HIV/AIDS in Nigeria. All names of persons are fictitious. Any resemblance to people, living or dead, is coincidental.

This book is divided into two parts. The first part consists of chapters 1 to 20. The second part is the notes taken in the interviews that I conducted with American-based Nigerian women who are permanent residents of the United States of America. The women expressed their lived experiences of polygamy and their perception of HIV/AIDS while practicing polygamy. In their own words, they expressed fear, helplessness, and disgust to polygamy, but they submitted that they used coping skills such as hope and prayer to live a life that their culture carved out for them.

# CHAPTER 1

I am a product of polygamy, not by marriage but by birth. My father had four wives who lived together with him and the children, including me. Three of the wives gave birth to the children, while one did not have a child with my father. The inability of the wife not to have a child was not by choice. According to her, it did not just happen. She always made this point known to my siblings and myself, even though I was very young at that time. We believed her because we know that, in Africa, it is the pride of the woman to have a child in marriage. A married woman without a child is a nonentity in the society and within her family circle. At the demise of the husband, the wife with no child has no inheritance. The husband's family members drive some women with no children out of the home, or the women leave of their own free will after the husband's death, as is the case with my father's wife who had no child with him and left of her own free will after my father's death.

I did not experience much of polygamy because my father died when I was four years old. Three of his four wives, including my mother, were living together in his house in Ibadan before the first wife relocated to Lagos to be with her daughter, my oldest half-sister. While I was growing up, I saw a blend of sweet and sour relationships among my mother and the other wife. One time they were friends; another they were quarreling and calling each other names while spitting out their bitter experiences with each other when their husband (my father) was alive. Their young children took sides with their mother while the older ones tried to settle the quarrels. The side I took was that of amusement, confusion, and interest in the stories. I wanted them to talk more about their bitter experiences of jealousy, competition, and intimidation while they lived with my father as his wives. I discovered that, when the wives were not fighting, they would say interesting stories about their encounter of polygamy. Usually they talked about my father being a good husband who took care of his wives by making sure there was money and food in the house for the family. Each of them accused him of loving the other one more. Sometimes my mother claimed that he loved her more. My siblings from the other wife said their mother also usually told them she was loved more than the other wives were.

Contrary to what I experienced in the relationship among my siblings and me, rivalry and squabbles among children of polygamous families were rampant. I heard stories from friends and witnessed a few. On one occasion while I visited a friend, her mother was fighting a co-wife because the co-wife had given more portion of the meal to her own child. As the child was flaunting the meal in the face of the other child, who was my friend's brother, my friend's mother took the meal from him and gave some of it to her son. The co-wife got mad, and a fight ensued. Each child sided with his mother. It turned to a huge fight. I learned later that, for several days, the children of both wives were fighting one another. When the fight became unbearable, their father left the house and did not come back until the wives found him after several days of searching and pleading with him to come back.

This incident is an example of disharmony that came with polygamy when I was growing up. It was always chaos in many polygamous homes with numerous children. It was rumored that many children of polygamous marriages do not belong to the father. The reason attributed to this is infidelity on the part of the wives who cannot be sexually satisfied by the husband because there are many wives. Infidelity, it was reported, is usually a two-way thing in polygamy. As the husband seeks more wives to boost his morale as "the man," the wives secretly seek a younger man to give them the intimacy and attention deprived in the home. Attention; money; distribution of food, house chores, or property; show of love (to wives or children); child education; the birth of a male child; and extended family interference are some of the things that caused quarrels in polygamous homes. I was fortunate not to experience the disharmony because my father died when I was very young.

The culture of marriage in Nigeria embraces extended family members called in-laws, who have much power and influence over the home to the extent that they can set the rules. Wives can be sent out of the home or totally divorced at the insistence of in-laws. Wives who wanted to remain in the house and enjoy their marriage always court the favor of in-laws, especially the mother-in-law.

One unforgettable story that my mother told me was about the time when my father married the fourth wife. They were all sharing a room as a family. When my father and his new wife wanted to have intimacy, the other wives were to pretend they were sleeping and also ensure their children were kept quiet, else they would be labelled jealous wives and scolded for their jealousy displayed by disturbing or allowing their children to disturb the husband's enjoyment of his new wife.

My mother said, "That was the system in those days. We had to adhere to it." She said further, "Thankfully your dad was a nice man. He would have married two women together at the same time and have intimacy with them together in the presence of other wives as a form of punishment." Again she said that was the system and other men were doing it to punish their wives. There was nobody to report to. The husband's word was law.

Then I got curious. I wanted to know the experiences of other women whose husbands were either good or bad. What could have kept them in that kind of marriage? Was love existing at all? What were their risks for sexually transmitted diseases (STDs)? Were they aware of the risks? What preventive measures for STDs did they take?

# CHAPTER 2

My interest in polygamy, a culturally acceptable marriage norm in Nigeria, bears the essence of this book. As I grew up seeing people practicing multiple partner relationships and hearing stories from my mother and siblings about polygamy, my interest grew.

Polygamy is rampant in Africa, and it is a system of marriage that is practiced in Nigeria (Doosuur & Arome 2013). It is culturally accepted for Nigerian men to have more than one wife and engage in sexual relationships with more than one woman. In African society as a whole and Nigerian society in particular, this is a show of wealth and power (Anyanwu 2013). Polygamy dates back to ancient times when men showed off their wives and concubines as a sign of wealth (Doosuur & Arome 2013).

Polygamy also has significance in men's work as farmers. Traditionally, having many wives and children made it possible to pursue farm work. Gradually polygamy became the way by which men could show their wealth and possessions (Doosuur & Arome 2013). Rich men, because they hold the power conferred by economic means, are free to have numerous girlfriends, usually young sex workers looking for means of livelihood in order to pay for school fees and help their families.

The belief of many rural dwellers is that polygamy, multiple partners, and gender inequalities are cultural ideas that have remained with the society, as they have been passed down from generation to generation. Through education and exposure to other cultures, Nigerian women have become empowered to reject or change the traditional belief that they are subject to the will of men and can be used to satisfy sexual urges.

# CHAPTER 3

Researchers have revealed that high-risk sexual behaviors such as polygamy facilitate the spread of HIV/AIDS. The CDC (2012) reported, "Multiple sex partners and/or infection with another sexually transmitted disease, such as syphilis, gonorrhea and chlamydia increase the risk of an HIV infection." A Joint United Nations program on HIV/AIDS (UNAIDS) report in 2012 estimated that global HIV/AIDS incidence was 35.3 million. According to the report, there had been 2.3 million new HIV infections globally in 2011, which represented a 33 percent decline in the number of new infections compared to 2001, when there had been 3.4 million.

Similarly, the number of AIDS-related deaths was also declining, with 1.6 million AIDS deaths in 2012 compared to 2.3 million in 2005. The target of UNAIDS is to halve HIV/AIDS transmission by 2015.

Despite the various steps that have been taken in terms of interventions of prevention and medication toward this target, significant challenges remain. Although there was a 50 percent decrease in new HIV infections among adults and adolescents in twenty-six countries between 2001 and 2012, other countries are far behind in pursuing the goal of reducing sexual HIV transmission by half.

According to the UNAIDS report, "Although trends in sexual behaviors in high-prevalence countries have generally been favorable over the last decade, recent surveys in several countries in sub-Saharan Africa have detected decreases in condom use and/or an increase in the number of sexual partners" (4).

The cultures of the sub-Saharan African countries have basic commonalities. The cultural practice pertaining to marriage in rural Nigeria, as in other African countries, is predominantly polygamous. HIV/AIDS interventions have brought awareness to the residents of urban areas, encouraging them to refrain from having multiple sexual relationships and engaging in polygamy. However, rural residents do not enjoy the benefits of such interventions because of their deep-rooted cultures.

According to AVERT (2014), an international HIV and AIDS charity, Nigeria has a population of approximately 166.6 million people, and an estimated 3.1 percent of the population is living with HIV and AIDS. In 2009, it was estimated that there were 220,000 AIDS-related deaths in Nigeria. In 2010, the life expectancy was lowered from fifty-four years for women and fifty-three years for men to an average of fifty-two years for both (AVERT 2011). The first cases of HIV/AIDS were identified in 1985, but the government did not respond to increasing transmission rates until 1991. At that time, the infection rate was 1.8 percent of the population. Rates climbed during the 1990s, rising to 3.8 percent in 1993 and 4.5 percent in 1998 and then increasing further to 5.8 percent in 2011 (AVERT 2011).

Efforts to deal with the HIV/AIDS epidemic in Nigeria became a priority of the Nigerian government in 1999, but in

2006, statistics showed that only "10 percent of HIV-infected women and men were receiving antiretroviral therapy (ART) and only 7 percent of pregnant women were receiving treatment to reduce the risk of mother-to-child transmission of HIV" (AVERT 2011).

The main HIV transmission route in Nigeria is heterosexual sex, which accounts for 80 to 95 percent of HIV infections (AVERT 2011). It is culturally accepted for Nigerian men to have more than one wife and engage in sexual relationships with more than one woman. In African society as a whole and Nigerian society in particular, this is a show of wealth and power (Anyanwu 2013). According to the CDC (2012), "Multiple sex partners and/or infection with another sexually transmitted disease, such as syphilis, gonorrhea and chlamydia increase the risk of an HIV infection."

# CHAPTER

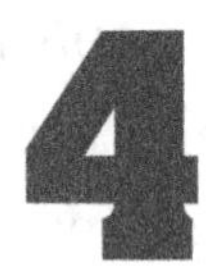

HIV/AIDS is recognized as a major problem in Nigeria, but there are gaps in HIV/AIDS health education initiatives. Most of these efforts have been focused on the major cities because of cultural sensitivities in rural areas (Obire, Nwakwo, & Putbeti 2009). Obire et al. (2009) further revealed that high levels of illiteracy and stigma are factors leading to concealment of HIV status among rural people. Although the HIV infection rate in Nigeria is low (3.6 percent) compared to other countries in West Africa such as Cameroon (5.3 percent) and Gabon (5.2 percent), it still equates to 3.4 million people with HIV (UNAIDS 2012). Additionally Nigeria is the most populous country in sub-Saharan Africa and has the highest number of immigrants in the United States (UNAIDS 2012).

Various contributing factors are associated with the spread of HIV/AIDS. Since the first outbreak of the virus, information has been gathered and studied regarding all facets of the disease, in an attempt to find methods by which to combat it either through prevention or medicine. According to Winn et al. (2006), HIV is one of the most devastating plagues facing humanity in the twenty-first century. It is changing societies and destroying lives, especially in the Third World. Nigeria, a country in southwest Africa that is one of the most populous countries of sub-Saharan Africa, has a high prevalence of HIV/ AIDS.

According to UNAIDS (2012) reports, 3.4 million people in Nigeria are HIV-infected. Through trade and travel, rural dwellers are beginning to encounter a greater incidence of HIV. In addition, rural dwellers are more rooted in a culture that promotes polygamy and multiple sexual partners, as well as male dominance in sex encounters.

Nigerian culture affords men the authority to determine the terms of sexual encounters. The belief of many rural dwellers is that polygamy, multiple partners, and gender inequalities are cultural ideas that have remained with the society as they have been passed down from generation to generation. Polygamy dates back to ancient times when men showed off their wives and concubines as a sign of wealth (Doosuur & Arome 2013). Polygamy also has significance in men's work as farmers. Traditionally, having many wives and children made it possible to pursue farm work. Gradually polygamy became the way by which men could show their wealth and possessions (Doosuur & Arome 2013). It is customary for a woman to remain married despite experiencing abuse.

According to Nigerian tradition and in present-day relationships, if a wife desires to avoid losing her husband or partner, she cannot demand that the husband use a condom during sexual encounters or ask for testing for HIV before intimacy (Doosuur & Arome 2013). Poverty adds its own share to this phenomenon. Men are richer than women are, causing disparity between the sexes, due to a cultural tradition of women not working. Most women are not allowed to work in Nigeria; therefore, wives are caregivers of children.

The culture in rural areas favors polygamy to a greater extent than the culture in urban areas, where education and exposure have afforded women the opportunity to stand for themselves. Nigerian women who immigrate to the United States fall into this category.

In my interaction with Nigerian immigrant women who married into polygamy before leaving Nigeria for the United States, I conducted interviews and looked into the lived experiences of polygamy as these women experienced. The participants of the interview were ten Nigerian immigrant women who married into polygamy in Nigeria but were, at the time of the interview, living in the United States, either in single-partner relationships or as single mothers. They were interviewed to share their lived experience of polygamy and their perceptions concerning how polygamy affects HIV/AIDS.

During the interview, the women were no longer practicing polygamy and resided in the United States as citizens or permanent residents. The interview was conducted in an effort to understand the role that polygamy plays in the spread of HIV/AIDS. According to Do and Meekers (2009), women are more likely to report their risk of HIV/AIDS when they are aware of their husbands' or partners' sex escapades. A UNAIDS (2010) report from the National HIV/AIDS and Reproductive Health Survey (NARHS, 2007) indicated that more females (4.0 percent) than males (3.2 percent) were infected with HIV in Nigeria.

Researchers who studied HIV/AIDS or polygamy used focus groups to interview both men and women as a group or women residing in Africa, a method that is likely to influence women's responses. The goal of this interview was to collect information from these women in order to determine what is needed to develop preventive interventions for women in polygamy so as to reduce the prevalence of HIV/AIDS. In addition, this exercise provides information to educate members of the younger generation in order to dissuade them from becoming involved in polygamy and multiple sexual relationships.

# CHAPTER

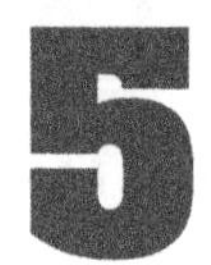

## Polygamy in Nigeria

### The Structure of Polygamy and Its Criticisms

The structure of polygamy involves one central spouse having multiple partners, which obviously yields two inequalities (Strauss 2012). The central spouse exerts greater control over the larger family. Normally, the central spouse dominates the family in terms of meeting expectations and roles of other family members. There are multiple forms of polygamy. *Polygyny* occurs when a man marries multiple women, while *polyandry* refers to one woman marrying multiple men (Strauss 2012). On the other hand, *polyamory* refers to informal sexual relationships among individuals of both sexes that may or may not involve marriage (Strauss 2012).

In some communities, both polygyny and polyandry may be practiced along with less formal sexual relationships; thus, the umbrella term *polygamy* is adequately used to refer to any and all of these various forms of multiple-partner relationships. While Strauss (2012) asserted that polygamy should be sexually and gender-neutral, in Nigeria, polygamy is only practiced by men in the family. The reason for this singular form of polygamy is that this behavior has long been the culturally and socially accepted norm.

While many scholars claim that polygamy creates gender inequality, there is a lack of sufficient data on this matter. The notion that polygamist communities condone family and spousal abuse is generally a misconception resulting from sexist culture of a particular society (Strauss 2012). Indeed both men and women in polygamist societies care for their spouses, children, and the wider family (Strauss 2012). However, it has been posited that it is only possible for traditional polygamy to be equal if both spouses can marry other spouses within and outside the family (Strauss 2012).

## Gender Roles in Polygamy

Culture is a vital aspect of everyday life of people. In Nigeria, every tribe has its own cultural and ancestral practices. Gender roles, family planning, and family structures vary greatly across tribes. For example, in the Kanuri tribe of northeastern Nigeria, men can marry up to four wives and rear an average of sixteen children (Mairiga, Kullima, Bako, & Kolo 2010). Kanuri women are expected to follow specific traditional family planning rules. These rules include adequate child-spacing, prolonged breastfeeding, and contraception using ornaments, spiritual invocations, and dried herbs (Mairiga et al. 2010). Northern Nigeria is Muslim-dominated, and there is a widespread practice of polygamy because the Islamic code provides for equal treatment and sustenance of all spouses (Ilevbare 2009).

In Nigeria, the size of a family is considered indicative of wealth (Anyanwu 2013). Several reasons have been posited for this:

1. The more wives a man has, the more political alliances he makes.
2. More wives yield more children, and children are considered essential to the household's workforce in generating household income (Anyanwu 2013).
3. Having many wives gives a man an increased sense of sexual gratification. Having multiple wives implies male dominance; whatever sexual needs a man has, he can have those needs met.

Some argue that polygamy provides greater reproductive health for women, who have time to rest after bearing a child because other wives are available to take her place laboring in the fields or tending to the other children.

# CHAPTER 6

## Overview of HIV/AIDS

HIV is a slow-replicating virus that weakens the immune system by destroying the T-cells or CD4 cells in the bloodstream. The primary function of these cells is to fight disease and infection (US Department of Health & Human Services [DHHS] 2014). There are three stages of HIV infection. These stages are dependent on factors such as age, HIV subtype, coinfection with other viruses, nutrition, stress, genetic background, ART, and the ability of the infected person to follow a doctor's recommended treatments (DHHS, 2014).

The first stage of HIV is the acute infection stage. This stage is characterized by symptoms such as fever, sore throat, rash, muscle and joint pains, and headaches. These telltale symptoms appear within two to four weeks after infection (DHHS 2014). At this stage, the virus reproduces rapidly within the bloodstream by using and ultimately destroying CD4 cells. At this stage, the risk of transmission is particularly high because high levels of the virus are circulating in the bloodstream.

Once the majority of CD4 cells have been destroyed, the virus enters the second stage, clinical latency, where the disease continues to develop but at a slower pace, and the symptoms present in the acute infection stage will have dissipated or disappeared entirely (DHHS 2014). Although infected people are symptom-free, they remain at high risk of transmitting the virus to others. Individuals who take ART may remain at the clinical latency stage for years or decades and are at lesser risk of transmitting the virus.

People in the clinical latency stage who do not seek treatment will eventually experience an increased viral load and significantly decreased CD4 cell count. When a person's CD4 cells fall below 200 cells per cubic millimeter, he or she is considered to have progressed to AIDS, the third stage of HIV (Kanki 2013). A person with AIDS is vulnerable to infections and infection-related cancers or opportunistic infections (DHHS 2014). Individuals with HIV who develop opportunistic illnesses are considered to have progressed to AIDS, despite having CD4 counts above 200 cells per cubic millimeter. The life expectancy of persons who progress to AIDS without treatment is from one to three years.

# CHAPTER 7

## History and Origin of HIV/AIDS

The first description of HIV/AIDS was published in the June 5, 1981, issue of *Morbidity and Mortality Weekly Report* by the CDC (De Cock, Jaffe, & Curran 2011). HIV is believed to have originated from nonhuman primates in sub-Saharan Africa and was communicated to humans at the turn of the twentieth century (Chavan 2011). A phylogenetic analysis of HIV and the simian immunodeficiency virus (SIV) of chimpanzees revealed that the cross-species transmission, or zoonosis, occurred early in the twentieth century; however, uncertainty remains about the circumstances behind the zoonosis (De Cock et al. 2011).

The most widely accepted theory regarding this zoonosis is the hunter theory, which posits that chimpanzee SIV was transferred to humans as chimpanzees were killed and eaten by hunters or when hunters' flesh wounds were infected by chimpanzees' blood (Chavan 2011; Wolfe et al. 2004). Although SIV is inherently a weak virus that the human immune system can suppress, the theory suggested that several rapid transmissions of the virus from one individual to another enabled the virus to mutate into HIV (Chavan 2011). Some theorists have suggested that this rapid transmission may have been a result of repeated use of unsterilized disposable plastic syringes with multiple patients, of which one or more may have had SIV (Katrak 2006).

Arguably the most controversial theory on the origin of HIV/AIDS involves the oral polio vaccine (OPV). According to this theory, it is posited that HIV can be traced to an OPV called CHAT that was allegedly harvested from kidney cells of SIV-infected local chimps (Katrak 2006). The CHAT vaccine was believed to have been administered to approximately 300,000 people in the former Belgian colonies of Africa, or present-day Democratic Republic of Congo, Rwanda, and Burundi.

However, recent analysis of the CHAT vaccine showed it had no trace of either HIV or SIV; rather the original developers of the OPV used macaque monkey kidney cells for harvesting, which could not have been infected by either virus (Berry et al. 2005). Other theorists continue to contest, debate, and test this theory, and controversy persists as more evidence from both sides of the debate continues to emerge.

A more recent theory is that of colonialism. The theory of colonialism is loosely based on the hunter theory and the contaminated needle theory, but it provides a more thorough and concise description of the circumstances surrounding the zoonosis. Proposed by an anthropologist and two postgraduate students, the colonialism theory indicates that the zoonosis can be traced to colonial practices in French Equatorial Africa and the Belgian Congo (Katrak 2006). During colonial rule, the African natives endured poor diets and sanitation, and they worked to exhaustion. The combination of lack of adequate resources, which forced doctors to reuse unsterilized needles and syringes, and a rampant sex trade contributed to undermining people's immune systems, making them more susceptible to infection (Katrak 2006). Thousands of laborers would have died before showing symptoms of AIDS, while those who showed symptoms would not have appeared any different from others who were infected with other diseases (Katrak 2006).

# CHAPTER

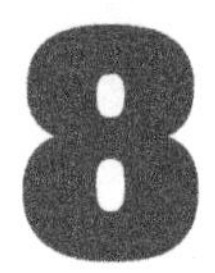

## Global HIV/AIDS

As HIV/AIDS continued to spread globally, national and international efforts were expanded to understand, prevent, treat, and educate people about the virus and the disease. In the United States, the CDC created a dedicated entity, the Division of HIV/AIDS Prevention (DHAP), tasked with the dual purpose of educating the public to prevent the spread of HIV and helping those who had already tested positive for HIV to live with the disease and gain access to antiretroviral treatment. The CDC and health departments of other countries have collaborated to build strong and sustainable programs to respond to the HIV/AIDS epidemic.

At the international level is the Joint United Nations Programme on HIV/AIDS, or UNAIDS, which was launched in 1996 to strengthen the global response to the disease led by the United Nations (Knight 2008). Experiments and research conducted under the auspices of UNAIDS are intended to improve the understanding of the disease, especially new infections and strains that develop as the virus is transmitted, and to design treatments to these new strains of the virus

(D'Angelo, Pollock, Kiernicki, & Shaw 2014). Such efforts have led to the development of and increased access to ARTs that allow people to live full lives without developing other diseases related to HIV.

UNAIDS maintains consolidated records of HIV/AIDS statistics globally, including number of infections, strains, and treatments provided to people living with HIV. According to the latest report released by UNAIDS (2013), approximately 35.3 million people are living with HIV globally. New HIV infections have dropped by 33 percent since 2001 (that is, only 2.3 million people became newly infected with HIV in 2012), a significant decrease from 3.4 million in 2001. Among children, the rate of infection dropped by 52 percent, with only 260,000 children newly infected in 2012, down from 550,000 in 2001 (UNAIDS 2013).

Improvements have also been made in the number of AIDS-related deaths. The greatest number of AIDS-related deaths reported per year occurred in 2005, when 2.3 million deaths associated with AIDS were recorded. This staggering number was reduced by 30 percent in the latest report from UNAIDS (2013), which indicated that only 1.6 million deaths from AIDS-related causes were reported worldwide. HIV/tuberculosis remains the primary cause of death among people living with HIV; however, the number of tuberculosis-related deaths has fallen by 36 percent since 2004 (UNAIDS 2013). Such improvements have resulted from increased access to care and enhanced ART.

As of 2013, approximately 9.7 million people living with HIV had access to ART in low- and middle-income countries, a number that represents approximately 34 percent of people eligible for treatment under the 2013 World Health Organization

(WHO) guidelines (UNAIDS 2013). Improved access to ART and heightened educational awareness programs worldwide were made possible by increased investments in HIV response and prevention programs (UNAIDS 2013).

# CHAPTER 9

## HIV/AIDS in Africa

Because the origin of HIV was traced to Africa, the number of people living on the continent with HIV is higher than in other parts of the world. More specifically, the majority (almost 71 percent) of all people in the world living with HIV reside in the sub-Saharan region of Africa (D'Angelo et al. 2014; Hajizadeh, Sia, Heymann, & Nandi 2014; UNAIDS 2013). Within this region, studies have revealed a greater prevalence of HIV/AIDS among individuals with higher socioeconomic status (Hajizadeh et al. 2014). This distribution stands in contrast to those in Swaziland and Senegal, where HIV/AIDS is concentrated among poorer individuals (Hajizadeh et al. 2014).

In other African countries, such as Kenya, Uganda, and Zambia, HIV/AIDS prevalence is greater among urban poor and rural rich adults (Hajizadeh et al. 2014). The concentration of HIV/AIDS among rural individuals of higher socioeconomic statuses and urban residents in sub-Saharan Africa, which is in contrast with other parts of the world, warrants further research to better explain and understand the factors that lead to or predict such statistics. Considerable research has been conducted regarding the prevalence of HIV/AIDS in the region, including assessment of the extent of the spread of HIV/AIDS, the role of politics and media in prevention and care, people's levels of understanding on the issue, how people are educated about the disease, and stigma and stereotyping surrounding the condition.

Because the majority of people living with HIV/AIDS are in sub-Saharan African countries, much global attention, policies, and funding have been allocated to the region (Smith, Ahmed, & Whiteside 2011). The HIV epidemic in this region has had tremendous long-term demographic and social impact on the population, and internal funding is inadequate to address the issue. Despite continuous funding from foreign governments and international organizations, there remains a great need to improve access to ART and management options for people living with HIV/AIDS, as well as to increase preventive measures such as training and education to minimize transmission (Nkhoma, Seymour, & Arthur 2013).

Perhaps the most common method by which people learn about developments, statistics, and availability of treatment for HIV/AIDS is through mass media, such as television news reports, newspapers, magazines, and radio. These mediums play a part in disseminating information about the disease and educating people about prevention, their options, access to medical attention, and the need for antiretroviral maintenance. Given the importance of the media in the fight against HIV/AIDS in sub-Saharan Africa, the media warrants scrutiny and monitoring to ensure that reporting is responsible and dissemination of information remains on point and accurate.

In a systematic analysis of the impact of press-state relations or media systems on HIV/AIDS news coverage in

African Anglophone newspapers, the contained democratic media systems in South Africa and Nigeria were found to allow for greater positive societal-level responses than repressive autocratic media systems in Zimbabwe and Kenya (D'Angelo et al. 2014). Contained democratic media systems are identified by the following characteristics:

1. Both public and private entities conduct broadcasting.
2. Newspapers are mostly privately owned because there are few state regulations on the press.
3. There is moderately high press autonomy and professionalism.
4. Newspapers are relatively unidentified with political parties (D'Angelo et al. 2014).

On the other hand, repressive autocratic media systems are characterized by the state owning and running all broadcasting and supervising both public and private newspapers, as well as low press autonomy and high political parallelism (D'Angelo et al. 2014).

In analyzing two examples of each of these two media systems, D'Angelo et al. (2014) discovered some differences with regard to coverage and information dissemination of HIV/AIDS news. Stories and articles emanating from contained democratic media systems focus on the government agencies that are responsible for addressing the social costs of HIV/AIDS. These articles often cite prevention campaigns as more efficacious than is made evident in repressive autocratic media systems (D'Angelo et al. 2014). The different news agendas of these two opposing media systems have implications for people's knowledge about HIV/AIDS disease transmission and prevention. Media content affects people's decisions, priorities, and lifestyle.

In the case of HIV/AIDS, these choices can be catastrophic, especially if facts are misrepresented and the public is misinformed. This study is expected to provide information to the Nigerian Ministry of Health on knowledge and attitudes relating to the spread of HIV/AIDS held by women who are affected due to their submissive role in polygamous marriage. This could give correct information that has been lacking in different types of mass media that may lead to adequate prevention and control of HIV/AIDS.

# CHAPTER 10

## HIV/AIDS in Nigeria

As part of sub-Saharan Africa, Nigeria has fought the HIV/AIDS epidemic since the early 1980s, when the disease was first described and recognized globally (Obidoa & Cromley 2012). Since those early days, the Nigerian Federal Ministry of Health has monitored the transmission of the disease and created programs and policies to address the epidemic. Although the rate of HIV/AIDS in Nigeria rose from 1.8 percent in 1991 to 5.8 percent in 2001, such efforts by the Ministry of Health, along with foreign and international support, reduced the prevalence to 5.0 percent in 2003, 4.4 percent in 2005, and 3.6 percent in 2012 (Obidoa & Cromley 2012).

Despite the decline in newly diagnosed cases, approximately 3.4 million people in Nigeria are living with HIV, and thousands of people are still at great risk of infection (UNAIDS 2012). Concerted efforts must be continued to increase access to ART, educate people on precautions against transmission, and improve living conditions to reduce risk of comorbidities associated with HIV/AIDS (UNAIDS 2012). Additionally there is a need to study the factors that promote the spread of this epidemic in the country and the region.

Researchers have explored the behavioral risk factors known to lead to the spread of the infection within a small sociogeographic area (Obidoa & Cromley 2012). Among the most cited reasons for the spread of HIV/AIDS in sub-Saharan Africa are the large population, high fertility rate, and inability to meet contraceptive needs, which protect against the transmission of sexually transmitted infections and HIV (Lawani, Onyebuchi, & Iyoke 2014).

Because of the high risk of infection, dual contraceptive methods (that is, the use of both condoms and another effective method) are encouraged among women, whether they are infected with HIV or not. However, a cross-sectional descriptive study of married HIV-positive women in Nigeria showed that most HIV-positive women lacked awareness about dual contraception methods (Lawani et al. 2014).

Of the 658 women surveyed, 447 (67.9 percent) lacked awareness of dual method use, and only 179 (27.2 percent) practiced it. Respondents cited lack of awareness and nondisclosure of their HIV status as the primary reasons for not using dual methods. The most common form of dual method reported was the combination of condoms and injectable hormonal contraceptives (Lawani et al. 2014). As expected, sexually transmitted infections and unplanned pregnancies were higher among women who did not use dual methods.

The behavior of both men and women toward consistent use of dual contraceptive methods is influenced by their awareness of HIV status and their decision to disclose their conditions to their partner. Despite improvements in treatment, there remains a stigma against HIV/AIDS, which hinders both prevention and treatment (Odimegwu, Adedini, & Ononokpono 2013). A cross-sectional random study of Nigerians revealed negative public attitudes toward HIV/AIDS-positive people, and this stigma is a strong predictor of voluntary counseling and testing (Odimegwu et al. 2013). Because of this widespread stigma, the likelihood of Nigerians pursuing voluntary counseling and testing is low, which consequently decreases the use of ARTs and the chances of survival (Odimegwu et al. 2013).

Prevalent negative attitudes about HIV/AIDS have serious implications for the epidemic in Nigeria and other countries. The success of national, foreign, and international efforts to address the AIDS pandemic through education, testing, and treatment are contingent upon the destigmatization of HIV/AIDS (Odimegwu et al. 2013). Hence, in addition to providing medical assistance and services to people living with HIV/AIDS, efforts must be made to educate the public and humanize HIV/AIDS-positive individuals such that people's perceptions about HIV/AIDS are improved.

Improving people's perceptions of HIV/AIDS and those living with the disease is believed to promote voluntary counseling and testing, as well as consistent use of precautions to avoid transmission and infection (Odimegwu et al. 2013). In Nigeria and several other sub-Saharan African countries, scholars and researchers have posited a link between polygamy and HIV/AIDS (Saddiq, Tolhurst, Lalloo, & Theobald 2010). Despite hypotheses regarding this connection, research conducted to date is inconclusive. The next section offers a brief discussion of polygamy in the Nigerian context and relates this behavior to vulnerability and resilience to HIV/AIDS.

CHAPTER

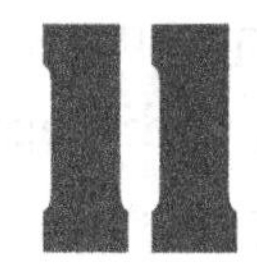

## Polygamy and HIV/AIDS in Nigeria

Polygamy is an institutionalized norm, not only in sub-Saharan Africa but also across the world. In some countries, polygamy is legal and allowed under common law. Islam, one of the widely practiced religion in Nigeria, supports the practice of having many partners in a marital union. In the United States, leaders of the Church of Jesus Christ and Latter Day Saints used to teach and practice polygamy or plural marriage from the midnineteenth century until 1890 (Hoyt & Patterson 2011).

Literature has documented that infidelity in polygamy promotes the spread of sexually transmitted diseases, including HIV/AIDS. Saddiq et al. (2010), in their qualitative study, posited that the practice of polygamy does not make people living in Nigeria vulnerable to HIV/AIDS; rather it is the social and cultural practices of the society to which the people belong. The practice of polygamy is a manifestation of the social relationships people can negotiate and experience. Polygamy socializes people similarly to the way in which institutions such as religion and education socialize people. Findings from focus groups and in-depth interviews with religious and community leaders and various groups of women and men in the community suggest that the religious institution in Nigeria greatly influences people's perceptions and attitudes about the practice of polygamy and the spread of HIV/AIDS (Saddiq et al. 2010).

The double standards of Nigerian men's extramarital relationships are rooted in the asymmetrical gender roles of the community. It is acceptable for men, but not women, to have more than one sexual partner. This phenomenon influences the spread of the disease because Nigerian women can acquire the disease from their sexual contact with their spouse, who might have acquired the disease from another wife or an extramarital relationship. The belief that men have greater sexual need and must be satisfied by their women put women at risk of sexually transmitted diseases.

Three themes emerged from Saddiq et al. (2010) study:

1. There is the perception of the relationship between polygamy and promiscuity. Promiscuity is associated with women whose needs—emotional, financial, social, or sexual—had not been met by their polygamous husband.
2. There is the role of religion in the perception and practice of polygamy. Some Muslim and Christian leaders consider the practice of polygamy as one way to fulfill religious obligations. Complications arise when the husband can no longer provide for the needs of his wives and children.
3. Women who engage in polygamy believe they are in competition with one another to gain the husband's favor. Co-wives sometimes engage in disputes with other wives and resort to looking for other men, which propagates the spread of the disease. This behavior promotes male dominance in Nigerian societies.

Women in Nigeria are expected to obey their husbands, whatever the circumstances may be. During the focus group discussions conducted by Saddiq et al. (2010), women reported recognizing sexual negotiations in their polygamous relationship. The women indicated that attempts at negotiation were perceived as bad behavior. Women who attempt to engage in sexual negotiations are constructed as promiscuous. When they request to have safe sex with dual methods, the husband will not consent. In most cases, the husband will accuse the wife of distrust and abandon her. Wives, out of fear of rejection, dare not question their husband's infidelity. Muslim leaders have stated that Islamic law does not prohibit sexual negotiations, but husbands perceive the law differently.

Furthermore, a study by Nyathikazi (2013) examined the relationship between HIV/AIDS and polygamy and the belief system and awareness of people when it comes to risk of infection as they practice multiple sex relationships. The study was done through focus group discussions among practicing male polygamists. Nyathikazi indicated that people practicing multiple sex relationships and polygamy might be at high risk for HIV/AIDS infection. The knowledge of the risk of infection did not prevent the respondents from having sexual relationships with multiple partners.

The study posits, among other things, that infidelity, not polygamy, is the factor that aggravates the spread of the disease. Where the man cannot sexually satisfy his numerous wives, the women go outside the marriage to look for sexual gratification. Again the issue of gender inequality plays a part in the nature of sexual practices, underscoring the need for further HIV/AIDS education. In this way, different institutions serve as mechanisms to mobilize and train different communities (Nyathikazi 2013).

HIV/AIDS is a global health problem. Although treatment exists, no cure has yet been found. Awusi and Anyanwu (2009) conducted a study to investigate and understand the perceptions and attitudes of pregnant Nigerian women toward HIV/AIDS. Findings suggest that most (91 percent) of the women are aware of HIV/AIDS and that the disease can be transmitted sexually (95.6 percent) and through infected blood (57.7 percent). While these women understand how they can become infected, their knowledge does not extend to prevention and treatment. For example, the women did not know the disease could be transmitted through breast milk (36.8 percent) and from mother to child (27.5 percent) through blood, both before and during birth. Fear of the disease was apparent in the study, with 95.6 percent of these women stating they would not want to stay in the same house as someone infected by the disease and 93.3 percent stating they would not care for a relative with AIDS.

From these findings, it can be inferred that poor knowledge or communication about HIV/AIDS status may also affect relationships and social behaviors with other people who are infected by the disease. Having knowledge about the nature of the infection reduces the stigmatizing effect of those surrounding the HIV/AIDS-positive individual.

Sub-Saharan African cultures have basic commonalities. The cultural practice of marriage in Nigeria, as with other African countries, is predominantly polygamous. According to Bowen (2013), there is the interplay between the universalist side of human rights advocacy and the culture-bound tradition in Ghana when it comes to understanding the nature of polygamy. Bowen examined the traditional polygamous marriage in the context of the legal system in Ghana, West Africa.

# CHAPTER 12

## Interventions for the Spread of HIV/AIDS

Efforts to confine the epidemic in Nigeria became a priority of the Nigerian government in 1999, but in 2006, statistics showed that only "10 percent of HIV-infected women and men were receiving ART and only 7 percent of pregnant women were receiving treatment to reduce the risk of mother-to-child transmission of HIV" (AVERT 2011). Nigeria has the second-largest population of people living with the disease worldwide (AVERT 2014). Even the younger ones in Nigeria are becoming vulnerable now to the spread of the disease. The three main HIV transmission routes in Nigeria were identified as heterosexual sex, blood transfusions, and mother-to-child transmission (AVERT 2014). At-risk groups include brothel and nonbrothel-based female sex workers, men who have sex with men, and injecting drug users (AVERT 2014).

The Ministry of Health of Nigeria Foundation for AIDS Care, Prevention and Advocacy, established in 2011, has a singular mission, to provide financial and technical support for the reduction of the spread of the disease. As part of its role in the battle against HIV/AIDS, the foundation is involved in provision of treatment and education at the grassroots level of the community through engagement and mobilization (AIDS Healthcare Foundation, 2012).

Sexual abstinence is a realistic intervention being considered by Nigeria to address the spread of HIV/AIDS infection (Aderemi & Pillay 2013). Young people's increased awareness and knowledge of how the disease is transmitted and prevented may have a positive impact. Condom promotion has encountered religious, social, and economic obstacles. Aversion to condom usage seems to be the real challenge for the Nigerian social context in terms of increased support for access to contraceptives to prevent the spread of HIV/AIDS infection (Audu, El-Nafaty, Bako, Melah, Mairiga, & Kullima 2008; Okulate, Jones, & Olorunda 2008).

Rather than intervening from a scientific perspective, religious institutions serve to educate men who practice polygamy on the need to observe good behavior, principally on how to treat women (Green 2011; Saddiq, Tolhurst, Lalloo, & Theobald 2010). Although women are typically placed in a subordinate position in Nigerian culture, religion and culture are not valid excuses for poor treatment at the hands of men. Nonetheless, the traditions, norms, and practices of society in Nigeria are connected to women's vulnerability for infection (Ostrach & Singer 2012).

Rural information programs are an important mechanism in the dissemination of quality information. These programs, however, suggest that information is shared equally between both sexes. The culture of violence propagated by the nature of polygamous relationships, including the spread of HIV/AIDS, cannot be overcome with information alone. People wish to do what they have always done. This behavior is indicative of Nigerians' strong attachment to cultural practices (Attah 2013).

Doosuur and Arome (2013) found men are more likely to perceive having contracted HIV/AIDS from women than are women to blame the men for infecting them. It may be possible to change the cultural aspect of this society and hence improve the well-being of women (Ugwokwe 2014). Doing so would likely eliminate or at least reduce the harmful practice of polygamy (Ugwokwe 2014; Ostrach & Singer 2012).

This change can be achieved with the aid of professional organizations such as the Federation of Female Lawyers in Nigeria, a women's and children's rights organization, and religious institutions (Akoto 2013). The organizations could share the necessary information with women and educate them on the consequences of cultural practices that put women at risk and how to avoid or at least mitigate those risks. Information can be passed through various cable formats. Children's libraries could serve as information centers to educate and train the next generation of men and women from an early age on the importance of gender equality and prevention of HIV/AIDS transmission through safe behaviors, including monogamous relationship (Ugwoke 2014). Similar actions conducted in urban settings have raised awareness of HIV/AIDS interventions and enlightened urban dwellers to refrain from multiple sexual partners and polygamy (Ugwoke 2014).

# CHAPTER 13

## Demographics of Respondents

My work as a public health researcher has afforded me the opportunity to talk to women who have experienced polygamy on their opinions regarding polygamy and HIV/AIDS in Nigeria. These women have left the shores of Nigeria without their husbands and are living as permanent residents and citizens in the United States of America. The respondents' ages at marriage were in the range of sixteen to twenty-one. Their husbands' ages at marriage were between twenty-one and fifty-five. While in Nigeria, some of their husbands were traders, one was a schoolteacher, and others were rich businessmen. Two of the women were assisting their husbands in their trades, one was a schoolteacher, one was a hairdresser, one was a nurse assistant, one was a school clerk, and four were housewives. The participants shared the same ethnic background, language, and culture. All spoke Yoruba, their ethnic language, and English. All reported having lived in rural Nigeria under a polygamous marriage with the man being the head and dictator to four to six wives of different ages. They added that there were numerous children to these marriages; however, according to tradition, other women's children were not counted. Additionally all reported ending participation in polygamy upon immigration to the United States.

Table 1

*Participants Demographics (Names are fictitious)*

| *Code (pseudonym)* | *Age* | *Years as immigrant in the United States* | *Marital status* | *Total education* | *Occupation in United States* | *Years married in Nigeria* | *Years married in the United States* |
|---|---|---|---|---|---|---|---|
| P1 (Aduke) | 42 | 10 | Married | College | Health | 14 | 8 |
| P2 (Alake) | 40 | 9 | Married | College | Health | 13 | 6 |
| P3 (Ajoke) | 39 | 6 | Married | College | Health | 12 | 5 |
| P4 (Ada) | 39 | 6 | Married | College | Health | 12 | 5 |
| P5 (Aminat) | 41 | 7 | Married | College | Health | 13 | 6 |
| P6 (Amoke) | 18 | 1 | Formerly married; in relationship | High school | Unemployed | 1 | 0 |
| P7 (Adanma) | 45 | 5 | Widow | High school | Business | Over 20 | 0 |
| P8 (Arike) | 30 | 4 | Married | College | Health | 6 | 3 |
| P9 (Agbeke) | 34 | 3 | Married | College | Health | 10 | 1 |
| P10 (Abike) | 45 | 4 | Married | High school | Business | Over 20 | 2 |

**Note:** "Years married in Nigeria" refers to years in a polygamous marriage.

Only one participant had more than one marriage. Her first husband died of HIV/AIDS. She is listed as formerly married, for she left her first husband, whom she married at age sixteen when he was fifty-five, after one year when she won the American visa lottery and self-identifies as single in a new relationship.

Respondent 1 got married in Nigeria at the age of eighteen

years to a man who was twenty-four years old. It was her first marriage. In Nigeria, she had a high school education. Her occupation in Nigeria was hairdressing. Her husband taught in the local primary school. Her husband had three other wives who were younger than she was. She was the first wife. The last wife was nineteen years old when her husband married her. She had four children with her husband in Nigeria. All of her children are with her in the United States.

Respondent 2's marriage in Nigeria began when she was eighteen and her husband was thirty-five years old. Her husband had no education, while she had a high school diploma. Throughout her marriage in polygamy, she was a housewife while her husband was engaged in business. Her husband had six other wives who were younger than she was. She was the third wife and had four children with her husband. One of her children is in United Kingdom. The remaining three are with her in the United States.

Respondent 3 got married into polygamy as the second wife at the age of twenty-one to her husband, who was twenty-seven and a trader like herself. They both had a high school education. She had three children in polygamy before relocating to the United States with her children. Her husband in Nigeria had two other wives whose ages she did not know.

Respondent 4 happens to be one of the few girls who went to high school where she lived while growing up in Nigeria. She married her husband in Nigeria when she was twenty-one years old and he was twenty-three years old and teaching at the local primary school. It was her first marriage, and she was the first wife. They both had a high school education. While the husband was teaching, she was a housewife. Her husband had three other wives who were younger than she was. She had four children with her husband in Nigeria. All four children live in Nigeria.

Respondent 5 married her husband in Nigeria when they were both twenty-one. It was her first marriage, and she was the first wife. Both had a high school education. While she was a ward maid (nurse assistant) in a hospital, her husband was a hospital clerk at the same hospital. There were two other wives in the marriage, but one died. She had four children with her husband in Nigeria. Two of her children reside in Nigeria, and two are in the United States.

Respondent 6 got married to her husband in Nigeria when she was sixteen and he was fifty-five years old. She did not finish high school in Nigeria, and her husband was illiterate. She was a housewife, while her husband was a very rich businessman. Her marriage to her husband in Nigeria was her first, and she was the last wife. She had no children and had four co-wives who were all older than she was.

Respondent 7 is a businesswoman who did not complete a high school education in Nigeria but got her GED in the United States. Her husband in Nigeria had a primary school education and started a lucrative transport business while she was a housewife. When they got married, she was nineteen years of age, and her husband was twenty-one. She was the first wife and had one child. She had five co-wives who were all younger than she was. Her husband died of AIDS. She lives with her child in the United States.

Respondent 8 got married to her husband in Nigeria when she was twenty years old and he was thirty-three. While in Nigeria, she had a high school education and worked as a school clerk while her husband was a teacher. She had three co-wives who had four children each. She was the third wife. She was one of the two participants who mentioned the number of children that her co-wives had. Others declined because, according to their cultural belief, no one counts other people's children. She had no children with her husband in Nigeria, who died of AIDS.

Respondent 9 got married to her husband in Nigeria at the age of twenty-one. Her husband, who was a trader like she was, was also twenty-one. Both had a high school education. It was her first marriage, and she had three children in the marriage. She had two co-wives who had three children each. She was the first wife. All of her children are in Nigeria. She was the other participant who mentioned the number of children that her co-wives had in polygamy.

Respondent 10 got married to her husband in Nigeria when she was twenty years old and he was forty. It was her first marriage. While she went to a teacher training school and became a teacher, her husband had a high school diploma and became a successful businessman. She was the second wife with two co-wives. She had six children with her husband in Nigeria. Three of her children are in the United States, and one lives in Canada. The rest are in Nigeria with her family.

# CHAPTER 14

## How Women Described HIV/AIDS

** All names are fictitious*

**Killer Disease:** All participants responded that they were well aware that HIV/AIDS is a "killer disease." All of them used this term. When I probed further how the term emerged, each responded, "through the TV and radio." They stated that the mass media were using advertisements in the form of drama, poetry, and songs to inform people about HIV/AIDS. Aduke stated that she did not take HIV/AIDS seriously until she saw people grow very sick and die from it. She claimed that people were dying so much of HIV/AIDS that it became a song in the village where she lived.

Alake said she had a friend who died of it, alongside her second child and husband.

> When my friend had the first child, she was fine, but the second child was a different story. The child started feeling sick all the time. They thought it was sickle cell. When they took him to the hospital, they discovered he had HIV. Then

> they tested all the other members of the family and discovered that it was only the first child that was negative. The husband was a bus driver who was going on tour for days. Who knows which of them had been having extramarital affairs?

All other participants claimed they either saw or heard about many people dying of HIV/AIDS. Adanma stated, "At first we thought it was a disease of the city people because we were hearing about people dying of it in the city. Later, we started seeing people around us in the village dying of AIDS."

She said hospital officials in the big cities were reporting HIV/AIDS as a "killer disease" anytime they gave news of death to a family.

**Sexual Transmission:** All participants stated that, at the time they were practicing polygamy, they thought the only means of transmission was by sex. Agbeke said, "We heard, if you have sex with a carrier, you will get infected and die soon." Abike stated, "Once you have sex with a prostitute, you catch it, and as a man with many wives, you get home and spread it to your wives."

Participants believed that prostitution was one of the means by which HIV/AIDS was transmitted sexually. In response, according to Ajoke, women attempted to reduce the amount of extramarital sex happening in their marriage. "I and other wives would fight our husband's mistresses and all the prostitutes around. We were doing that without our husband's knowledge."

When I asked how they were identifying and fighting the prostitutes, she responded, "We usually watch our husband secretly whenever he goes out, and if we see him often with any lady, we will know something is going on."

She stated further that they would go to prostitutes to warn them to leave their husbands alone, but if they did not stop, they fought them. She stated, "Young boys in the area also help us to fight them. By that, the prostitutes were running away from our area, and the mistresses were getting married."

Other participants also spoke about how prostitution declined because the wives were fighting prostitutes out of fear of HIV/AIDS. According to Amoke, "The prostitute business was not moving anymore in the village because the wives were fighting them."

Aminat indicated that she was always telling her children not to have sex because she feared they would catch HIV. Adanma responded that her fear was about her only child, who was "growing into a beautiful woman." She said, "I was always watching out for her. I didn't want the boys to come near her at all."

Amoke said her brother died of AIDS. "We never knew if he was having sex, but we suspected he was. How else could he have got it? That was the question then, but now I know better."

When I asked Amoke to clarify how she knew better, she explained that now she was surrounded by nurses who provide proper health education.

**Discrimination against People with HIV/AIDS:** All participants responded that people with HIV/AIDS were treated as outcasts. Alake stated, "Nobody would eat, play, or work with them, except their family members and their traditional healers that they go to when the hospitals reject them."

Agbeke said, "They were not giving HIV-infected people jobs and housing. Not even sitting with them. Their families are the ones who take care of them to the point of paying traditional healers for them."

Aminat stated, "Hospital workers don't accept them. They said they cannot cure them, and they were afraid of catching the disease too."

According to participants, hospitals in the village did not treat people with HIV/AIDS, unlike the hospitals in the big cities. They declared that people could not afford to go to the big cities resort to traditional medicine. When I asked if the traditional medicines cured HIV/AIDS, participants responded that the HIV-infected people who used traditional medicines eventually died within a short period of their diagnosis.

According to Ada, discrimination was the reason HIV/AIDS had spread so much in Nigeria. She stated, "People were not being sincere about their HIV status for fear of discrimination. Who doesn't want to live a normal life, like having a job, wives, and children?"

Arike added that her brother committed suicide because of fear of discrimination when he discovered that he had HIV. She said she was grateful to God that he was single, although other members of the family would have preferred that he had a child to live on after him.

# CHAPTER 15

## How Women Describe Polygamy

All participants believed that polygamy was one of the cultural behaviors responsible for the spread of HIV/AIDS. They all reasoned alike and admitted that a man cannot sexually satisfy all of his wives. Some participants (four out of ten) said this, in turn, resulted in the women secretly seeking satisfaction outside the family. According to these participants, though infidelity by women was not allowed, young women who could not get sexual satisfaction from their husbands had secret boyfriends with whom they satisfied themselves. According to them, this relationship was arranged by the wife, who looked for a young man in the community and asked him to be her boyfriend. They stated further that the wives gave gifts and money to their boyfriends to keep them quiet because, if their husbands or his relatives got to know about it, their marriage would be over. The secret, they stated, would be kept between the boyfriend and the wife.

According to Alake, "Many of the wives go outside for satisfaction and bring HIV with them. The husband will have sex with her and transfer it to other wives."

Amoke stated that she had a boyfriend outside her marriage because her husband was too old to satisfy her sexually.

Ajoke said, "The man outside the marriage with whom the woman satisfies her sexual urges surely must be promiscuous himself. He is therefore a carrier of STDs."

Aduke, who contradicted this, stated,

> I knew I was at risk, but women are usually faithful in marriage because it is against the culture for a married woman to be seen with another man, but the man is the one who brings HIV by sleeping with different women. There must have been a sexual relationship between them before he decided to marry her. Trust me. Polygamists go about sampling women in bed before marrying the most sexually active one. By so doing, they acquire and spread HIV.

Abike's interview provided yet another dimension to the issue, supporting Ajoke's view that women seek sexual satisfaction outside marriage. "Younger wives usually have sex with older children of their husbands if their husbands are too old to sexually satisfy them. They look for the one who looks very much like the husband so that, if they get pregnant by accident, the child will look like their husband and there will be no suspicion."

Though participants were divided in their opinion of who was more faithful in marriage, all participants believed that extramarital affairs actually occurred in polygamy and they were precursors to HIV/AIDS. Only one participant, Amoke, admitted indulging in extramarital affairs with her boyfriend in high school, whom she would have married if her marriage to her polygamous husband had not been arranged. They all admitted that, if a wife committed sexual immorality, it must have been lack of satisfaction by the man. They stated, however, that women were not allowed by tradition to have extramarital affairs.

Apart from Amoke, who stated that her co-wives liked her and she liked them too, participants did not have a good relationship with co-wives because there was suspicion of extramarital affairs and competition among wives to court the husband's favor. According to participants, the first wife had the most power by tradition, but the favorite wife of the husband assumed the most power. All admitted that they knew they were at risk of contracting HIV/AIDS. All also stated that the men were aware of the risk of HIV, but they considered their ego to be more important.

**Male Dominance:** The general consensus of participants was that women were subject to men in marriage. According to participants, the cultural tradition was for women to have no choice in anything concerning their lives, including decisions regarding the terms of sexual intimacy. In their responses, each displayed a general feeling of helplessness associated with HIV/AIDS and the polygamous lifestyle. All participants were well aware of their exposure to health issues but displayed a feeling of surrender to polygamy.

Ada stated, "Polygamy is terrible. What can we do? It is the culture that we were born into, and we women have been taught to accept that our husband will marry more than one wife."

According to participants, parents taught their children from childhood about the roles of husband and wife. The role of the husband was to be the decision maker and controller of the home while the woman was to be submissive to him and take care of him and the children.

Aduke commented about her husband, "He was the breadwinner and the head of the family. He was also the decision maker, and we had to obey him, whether his decision was good or bad."

Adanma reflected, "He was the head of the house, decision maker, and everybody feared him. He was the one responsible for providing the money that we all spent."

Alake recalled, "He was the breadwinner, and he was doing that very well. He always boasted that he is a superman because he was feeding many people in his house."

This perception was true even for women who were making their own money. They all expressed a feeling of security when their men had money.

**Quality of Family Unit:** Participants stated that, despite their perception of risk of contracting HIV/AIDS while in polygamy, the quality of family unit in polygamy undermined their perception. According to participants, all the members of the family lived in the same house and ate together. This, they stated, allowed their children to be in harmony. Though children sided with their mothers during quarrels, the older children quickly settled such quarrels so the home could be at peace. Participants described the wives' quarrels as mostly verbal and emanating from issues such as money, competition, other wives' children, and space. Participants believed that one of the struggles of polygamy was space.

According to Ada, "The children like it [polygamy] because they have many siblings to play with. The wives don't like it [polygamy] because they always fight over everything like other wives' children, money, space, etc."

Aduke described the struggles of polygamy by saying,

> We all had our different rooms. Each wife and her children live in one room separate from the husband. We all share same living room and eat together. In our house, we had two bathrooms and one kitchen. The only struggle we have with the bathrooms is when both are occupied and someone needs to go out urgently. He will have to wait and call on the person inside the bathroom to be quick. Anyone who didn't want to be delayed will have to wake up earlier than other people to use the bathroom. Children of multiple wives get along or quarrel, depending on the rules of the house and how properly the husband handles the affairs of the home. In my home, our children were good with one another until we, their mothers, start to fight. They take sides, but after the fight, they make peace with one another first and come together to settle their mothers.

According to participants, this sense of harmony enjoyed by their children in polygamy and the way quarrels among wives was settled by older children, make polygamy interesting. They reported that wives did not consider HIV/AIDS in this type of situation.

**Marriage Dynamics:** The dynamics of marriage was a topic that participants described in detail. According to them, marriage was a social institution binding different families together in a way that did not allow for anyone to perceive the effects of HIV/AIDS as they went into polygamy. All gave an insight into how marriage was constituted and what occurred after the marriage.

Describing the culture of marriage in details, Ada stated,

> It is either through a man meeting a girl and asking her to marry him and the parents will be notified or parents will get together and arrange for their children to meet. In both ways, the man has to pay a bride price before the girl can marry him. The man doesn't need to inform his other wives and children before marrying a new wife, and everybody knows that. The wife is married to the man forever, no divorce except if the woman has extramarital affairs. He will send her back to her parents and curse her. No man will marry her again. This is very rare. Men are the ones who can have extramarital affairs. Women are not allowed to.

Adanma also stated,

> When a woman finishes school from sixteen years upwards, men will be asking her out. They can go directly to her or go through her parents or from parents to parents. The parents of the man bring gifts to the parents of the girl. The man also gives gifts to the girl and takes her out. The parents fix the date for marriage, and the girl becomes a wife after the man pays her bride price or dowry and takes her home. If she has children, she will stay married to the man forever. If no children, she can be sent out or abandoned and replaced with

> another new wife. If all her children are girls, she and her girls will not inherit anything from the man when he dies.

**Women Are Accustomed to Polygamy:** All participants believed that polygamy was a marriage system with which women were familiar.

According to Aduke, "It is the system. It is not possible to stop the men. If anyone tries that, they are just promoting extramarital affairs."

Alake explained that girls were taught from childhood to expect that they would not be the only wife in their marriage. All participants admitted that their parents lectured them about the roles of husband and wife in polygamy. According to Ajoke, some women looked forward to it, "especially when they start to bear children, knowing that their husbands will definitely need to satisfy himself."

Ada declared that she had witnessed a man marry two wives at a time without any of the wives complaining. According to her, the marriage was well celebrated. She said, at that time, she felt it was the normal thing, but now it felt disgusting to her because it was like treating a woman as a property. Aminat said she received a thorough lesson on how to have a good relationship with her cowives. She stated further,

> Any woman who thinks her husband is not seeing another woman is deceiving herself. In fact, some women even prefer to choose the wife for their husbands so that the husband will not go and bring a woman who will be fighting them. I knew I was at risk of contracting HIV, but I was lucky that my husband allowed me to choose wives for him.

Amoke stated, "When I married a man as old as my father, I expected I would meet some wives there, and I knew I was not going to be the last one."

Adanma, Arike, and Abike said it was a "system thing" to which women had become accustomed. Agbeke stated, "Women already know that their husband will bring another wife as soon as possible, so they are prepared for it. Polygamy can never be done away with. It is like killing the men's ego. They will look for another way of doing it."

All participants said that their parents lectured them about polygamy and they grew up in it before getting married; therefore they were familiar with it.

**Men Are Polygamous by Nature:** All participants declared that men were polygamous by nature. According to them, this nature fueled their attraction to as many women as possible. Aduke stated, "There are many examples in the Bible, even though God made one man and one woman."

Ada believed that economic hardship forced men to abandon polygamy, but not in its entirety. According to her, some family members helped men who did not have the means to acquire wives.

Aminat declared that the nature of men was such that men would always look for women to satisfy their sexual urges.

When I asked her how she came about this theory, she responded, "It is a thing of pleasure to them. It boosts their ego. African men love to boast of their numerous wives."

In Agbeke's opinion, men were polygamous by nature because they did not get pregnant and society did not frown against their promiscuity. She said, "In some parts of Nigeria, it is the joy of the parents when their son has numerous wives. It shows that he is a real man. Do you know that parents even boast of it?"

**Marginalization of Women:** Participants were unanimous that women were treated as property. Aduke stated, "We are not treated as equals, so we cannot make decisions about anything, including sex. So we are at risk of anything."

Alake stated, "I knew I was at risk of HIV/AIDS, but my children were girls. A woman is not regarded as anybody. Also if a woman doesn't have a male child, she may be divorced. My children were all girls. I needed to have a male child. If not, he would send me and my children out of his house. Where would I go? I had to keep on with the marriage until I had a male child."

According to Ada, "I knew I was at risk for HIV/AIDS and other STDs, but I was just praying. What can I do? Women are not allowed to talk."

Other participants also mentioned having a male child as one of the reasons women stayed in the marriage. They explained that female children did not have a right to their father's property when he died. They added that, at the demise of the husband, family members drove away wives who had no male child. They either took the children or sent them away with their mothers. Participants also stated that, if a woman did not have a child or had no male child, the husband and his family were allowed to replace her with another wife. In such cases, at the discretion of the husband, the woman could remain in the marriage or be sent out. The children were either taken from her or sent away with her. The woman went back to her parents and could decide to have another husband or remain unmarried. According to participants, the value attached to male children that marginalized women without male children was enough to stay in the marriage despite their perceived risk of HIV/AIDS.

**Fear of Rejection by the Husband:** All participants

stated that they were afraid of being divorced or abandoned by their husbands if they made it known that they were aware of the risk of HIV in their polygamous marriage. Agbeke declared that she knew there was the risk of HIV/AIDS, but she could not handle being rejected by her husband if she dared bring up the idea of using a condom. According to her and other participants, a woman who asked her husband to wear a condom was asking for trouble. She would be regarded as unfaithful and disrespectful, and that was enough grounds for divorce.

The youngest of the participants, Amoke (age eighteen), said she got married at sixteen to a man who had four wives. The marriage lasted one year. She said she was in constant fear because there was too much competition among the wives. According to her, the competition ranged from sex to materialism to courting the favor of the husband. She said, when her husband would not use a condom, she could not complain for fear of being abandoned.

Adanma relayed a similar experience,

> My marriage was a perfect one until the wives started arriving year after year. Before long, I was forgotten. I couldn't complain. You know, women cannot say anything, but thank God that I didn't get HIV. My husband eventually came down with HIV and some of the wives too. Oh! God bless the children. I don't know what has become of them. I had to come over here with my only child that I had, for him, as soon as I had the opportunity. The wives were always fighting, and our husband would leave the house as a form of punishment for us. Sometimes he would go for weeks, and we would have to welcome him

> with open arms if we didn't want him to go back. What a shame! Thank God I am not in that mess anymore. He died a few years ago. I have since decided to remain single, even here in America, because I just cannot handle the emotional disturbance of being under the control of a man.

Many of the women stated that polygamy was more common in the rural communities despite the widespread awareness of HIV/AIDS as a killer disease. They attributed polygamy in the rural communities to lack of education and civilization.

According to Adanma, "People are not well educated and civilized in the village like in the city. The city people don't usually marry many wives because they live like the Western people, although, if they want, they can do it. Nobody will question them. Every African girl knows that polygamy can happen in her marriage at any time."

According to participants, in the rural areas, women were not allowed to remain unmarried into their midtwenties and thirties because they wished to get advanced education and career.

Aduke stated,

> Such women don't stay in the village because no man will want to marry them. They will be too civilized for the husband to handle. Except if they get a man who has advanced education like themselves, which is rare in the village, such women will stay unmarried for their lives, and that cannot happen in the village. They will be labelled as prostitutes, and other women will be fighting them away from their husbands. It will be a shame to their parents.

# CHAPTER 16

## How Women Coped in Polygamy

### No Use of Protection

All participants indicated they were not using protection when engaging in sexual intimacy with their husbands while in polygamy. They responded that, if they requested that their husbands use a condom, he would think they had been having an extramarital affair.

Aduke stated, "Except if you are ready for false accusation and divorce, you cannot demand protection. I was just taking antibiotics, but I was doing it secretly so that he would not send me out or accuse me of not trusting him."

When I asked her if she knew that antibiotics did not kill viruses such as HIV, she said she did not know at that time, but she knew now.

Aminat stated, "In my thirteen years of marriage to him, he never used condom. He always said he hated it like hell. That means to me that he has tried it outside the marriage. Inside the marriage, no wife dares mention [condom use]."

She disclosed that one of her co-wives was "sent packing"

because she requested that their husband use a condom before sex with her. "Our husband said she must have been using it [having sex] with other men."

Arike noted it was disrespectful to the man when his wife demanded protection for sex, "It is like telling the man that he has a disease."

According to participants, men did not believe they had STDs. In the event of an STD, the man would query his wives, even if they had been faithful to him.

Alake provided another dimension, when she stated, "That is the reason men have many wives. If a wife is pregnant or nursing her child, instead of using protection or going outside the marriage, he can satisfy himself with another wife."

Amoke stated that women often did not use a condom as they did not want to use contraception to prevent conception despite the risk of HIV/AIDS. "Though I was afraid of catching HIV, I was also looking to have a child with him."

Ajoke explained that some women sought alternatives to condom use to protect against HIV/AIDS,

> I was not using protection, but I had a cream that I was using to rub my body before intercourse. I got the cream from a witch doctor without my husband's knowledge. If he knew, he would kill me, but I am sure other wives were doing it too. I think it helped because I married him for twelve years and did not have HIV.

Ajoke expressed her belief in the efficacy of traditional medicine to prevent HIV/AIDS. I asked other participants to explain to me their belief about using traditional medicine for protection against HIV/AIDS. Seven participants said they did not believe that traditional medicine could prevent HIV/AIDS, but they believed it could cure other diseases.

After Ajoke's interview, I used probes in subsequent interviews to determine if participants used alternative prescriptions (for example, saw a witch doctor) for protection. Two of them talked about using a witch doctor prescription for protection because they suspected that their husbands were seeing a witch doctor as a preventative measure for HIV/AIDS.

## Fear of HIV/AIDS

Fear of HIV/AIDS was the common term that participants used to describe the state of their sexual relationship with their husbands. All stated that they were in constant fear of HIV/AIDS, but they could not do anything because society frowned against divorce and single women. According to them, a woman who was unmarried or childless was stigmatized; therefore, women had to stay in their marriage to avoid stigmatization and to bear children. Eight of the participants stated that their sexual relationship with their husband in polygamy elicited fear or psychological distress because they knew their husbands had been with someone else and might have been infected.

The remaining two participants stated that, though they feared HIV/AIDS, they trusted and loved their husbands because they were not promiscuous. This may contradict the earlier view expressed that all men were promiscuous (or, contrarily, that women who thought differently were in denial); however, the participants appeared to distinguish between promiscuity and polygamy, the latter of which was viewed as being faithful to multiple wives. These two participants also stated that they did not trust the other wives when it came to extramarital affairs.

Amoke noted, "The wives are the ones who bring in the disease."

According to Abike, at the early stages of her marriage, she did not fear much until the third wife arrived. "From the moment I saw her, I knew we were doomed. She was always talking and behaving like a prostitute. I don't know why my gentle husband married such a lousy slut. How we all escaped HIV/AIDS, I don't know 'til today, but I was always praying anytime my husband had sex with me."

## Plan for Sex

All the participants responded that sex was always planned. Each wife had her own day to sleep with the husband. Alake said sometimes they had a mix-up and the wives would fight the whole day. She stated further that the husband sometimes created the mix-up so as to sleep with the favorite wife.

Amoke stated, "This was the most frustrating for me."

Arike stated that, after some time, her husband did not include her in the plan anymore because she had no child. She added that, although she did not like that he abandoned her, she was grateful that she was not in fear of contracting HIV.

Ada explained by stating,

> Sex plan is a roster that we do to show who sleeps with him at what day of the week. It is something that we have to keep to; else it turns to a huge fight. Except the husband changes it. No wife can take another wife's position. It is rare for

> husbands to change it unless the wife requests for change due to illness or pregnancy. Pregnant and nursing wives don't participate at all.

Aminat explained planned sex better by stating,

> It is a roster that we make to show the days when each wife would sleep with the husband. When we were three, we used to make it a daily affair. My days were Mondays and Tuesdays, the second wife Wednesdays and Thursdays, and the third wife Fridays, Saturdays, and Sundays. The last wife usually has more days because she is the most recent wife and needs to enjoy the husband more. When the second wife died and our husband refused to marry another one to replace her, I took her Wednesdays, and the third wife took her Thursdays. When one of us is pregnant, nursing, or menstruating, it is enjoyment galore for the other wives because the wife is excluded from the roster.

Amoke also talked about the planned sex by stating,

> We had a roster for when to sleep with our husband. Each wife goes to sleep with him on her own day. At the time I came, the first wife was not participating in it because, according to our husband, she was too old for sex. Later I learned that she was abandoned because she asked our husband about condom and he started suspecting her. That left four of us for seven days.

> I got three days being the youngest and newest wife. The fourth wife had two days, and the rest had a day each. Any of us who was pregnant or menstruating would give up her place to one of the other wives.

## Be the Obedient Wife

According to all participants, the knowledge of HIV/AIDS could not prevent them from having sexual relationship with their husbands. The culture dictated that a woman must be obedient to her husband. According to them, they had no choice because culture forbid from women denying their husband sex or dictating when and how it was convenient for them. Participants stated that co-wives were always fighting, but when it came to dealing with their husbands, they had to carry out his orders. Participants considered obedience to their husbands as a self-defense mechanism to avoid their husbands' discipline. Participants reported that women who did not want to incur the wrath of their husbands were usually following their husbands' rules and demands for sex.

According to participants, in Nigeria, men could beat their wives for any offense without the wives beating the husband back or reporting him to anyone in the community. According to Adanma, "No, we don't go to anybody for support. What happens in the home stays in the home. That is one of the trainings we received as girls."

According to Ada, when the wife was injured from the husband's discipline, she could not call the police because the police would support the man and there was no law supporting the woman in the village. In large cities, there were priests and elders who acted as counsellors. The counseling was usually more about how the woman would be more obedient to the husband. According to participants, wives did not go to the hospital for treatment if injured by their husbands through discipline because the husband, who was the custodian of the money in the home, would not pay the hospital bill.

## Coping Skills

Coping skills came out as a common theme in polygamy where participants mentioned how they tried to find ways to protect themselves from getting infected as a result of having sex with their husbands. Seven of the participants reported to rely solely on prayers and hope, while three participants actually took additional measures such as playing sick and using cream from local traditional healers to protect themselves. In both cases, the participants indicated that the underlying fear and coping mind-set would negatively impact their sexual relationship.

# CHAPTER 17

## Escape to a New Life

Some of the participants won the American visa lottery, while others were invited to America by families who also helped them to get their permanent residency. They talked about their former husbands' willingness to release them because everybody heard about the good life in America. They stated that their former husbands allowed them, hoping they would help them (the husbands) to come to America too. The women stated that they saw the opportunity to come to America as a way of escape from polygamy, but they did not have the guts to tell their husbands. Participants talked about their new lives in America. All of them except Adanma had men in their lives. Amoke was not married but had a steady relationship with an African American man whom she described as loving her as much as she loved him.

Abike stated, "Anyway, my present husband is the best. I am free of fear, and I can talk. Thank God for America."

Ajoke described her present marriage, "It is heaven on earth. I thank God for bringing me here and meeting my present husband. My past marriage was a mess. My present husband is Nigerian too. He was born here and grew up here. He is a nurse. We spend our money together and love each other."

Alake remarked about her present husband,

> He is Nigerian. He came here when he was twenty years old. He is forty now and has two children with his late wife. I have a child with him. He is a teacher. He allows me to make my decisions, and he is never controlling. We spend money together. We raise our children together and go to places together. My children love him as their own father. He means everything to me.

The willingness of these women to share their experiences in polygamous marriages provided a window into their lives: the ubiquitous presence of polygamy in their culture; the dominance of men over women; the fear of HIV/AIDS; their helplessness to protect themselves from the disease; and their feeling of joy to escape to a new life where they are free from polygamy.

Another reason participants stated for staying in polygamy despite their perception of risk of HIV/AIDS was procreation. According to the women, a woman without a child faced discrimination.

It appeared that participants were not happy being in polygamy. As each narrated the history of her life in polygamy, each showed emotions of frustration and sadness. Conversely, each showed emotion of happiness as she talked about her new life and marriage in America.

# CHAPTER 18

## My Perspective

It appears that women from the rural areas of Nigeria have little information regarding the nature of the transmission of HIV/AIDS. When these women were practicing polygamy, they perceived HIV/AIDS as a killer disease that was transmitted through sex and carried stigma. Their knowledge at the time they were practicing polygamy did not demonstrate an understanding of other forms of HIV transmission such as breast milk, blood transfusion, lacerations, use of unsterilized syringes, and so on.

Lack of adequate information has been linked to the spread of HIV/AIDS (AVERT 2014). Studies have documented that, during the earlier days of HIV, people considered hand shaking, toilet seats, eating utensils, and mosquito bites as means by which HIV/AIDS could be transmitted (Obidoa & Cromley 2012; Odimegwu et al. 2013). This lack of information contributes to discrimination against people who have HIV/AIDS. Participants claimed that anyone with HIV/AIDS was avoided in the community and the hospitals did not accept them.

This attitude reveals perceived severity of the disease.

For this reason, people did not disclose their HIV status and consequently did not present for testing and counseling. Perhaps this lack of information is also the reason many people in Nigeria are not aware of available treatment such as ART, which has been approved for use to extend the lives of people living with HIV/AIDS. With the use of ART, people are beginning to live longer and manage opportunistic infections associated with the disease (DHHS 2014).

Stigma against people with HIV/AIDS is consistent with the cross-sectional study conducted by Odimegwu et al. (2013) discussed in the literature review. They revealed that public attitudes toward people with HIV/AIDS are a strong predictor of voluntary counseling and testing. Because of this stigma, the likelihood of Nigerians pursuing voluntary counseling and testing is low, which consequently decreases the use of ARTs and the chances of survival.

Another aspect of stigmatization reported by participants was discrimination against single women. The Nigerian culture looked down on single women of marriageable age and divorced women. According to the women, they were labelled as prostitutes. This was one of the reasons women marry and stay married despite perceived susceptibility to HIV/AIDS brought about by their promiscuous husbands or co-wives.

Alongside discrimination was the preference for male children. Where a woman had no male child, she cared less about infection despite perceived severity of the infection. This reveals that, if the woman were a carrier of infection herself, the desire to have a male child would override disclosing that she was a carrier.

Participants reported that there was a link between HIV/AIDS and polygamy. This showed that women who practiced polygamy had a high level of risk perception. All of them declared that polygamy fueled HIV/AIDS because of extramarital affairs, which existed in polygamy. Two participants stated that there was faithfulness on the part of their husbands, but the wives who had no sexual satisfaction by their husbands could not be trusted when it came to extramarital affairs.

This was in line with the observations made by Sadiq et al. (2010) and Nyathikazi (2013) in the literature reviewed. The researchers posited that extramarital affairs in marriage was what made polygamy a fuel to HIV/AIDS. Polygamy practiced according to the rule of faithfulness could not promote HIV/AIDS.

A study on women in polygamy will extend knowledge on the struggles that women who married into polygamy experienced in an attempt to adhere to culture. According to participants, Nigerian women had no voice or choice in anything pertaining to their lives. As they had no power to negotiate the terms of sex encounter, women were vulnerable to HIV/AIDS.

Participants reported constant fear of HIV/AIDS as they lived their lives in polygamy. It appeared that their lived experience of polygamy was tainted with fear of infection of HIV/AIDS, but the women had no power to free themselves from the culture of polygamy until after immigrating to the United States, where there was freedom of speech for women.

Participants believed the nature of men was that of polygamy and women were trained to accept this notion. This belief posed a high risk to contracting HIV/AIDS. In some parts of Nigeria, men could marry as many wives as they wanted. Men married many wives to satisfy their sex desire and to pass off as wealthy. In Nigeria, the size of a family was considered indicative of wealth (Anyanwu 2013). Though Ilevbare (2009) stated that the Islamic code allowed polygamy and equal treatment of wives, women who held the belief that men were polygamous by nature did not get sexual satisfaction from their husbands and consequently looked outside the marriage for satisfaction.

One of the participants declared that there were instances of younger wives cheating with older children of the husband. Another participant reported that she had a boyfriend because her husband, who was as old as her father, could not satisfy her sexually. From these reports, one could deduce that sexual relationship in polygamous marriage was a risky affair. The risk was more pronounced where men did not accept that they could be infected. When they got infections, they did not disclose it, and if they disclosed it, they blamed their wives for infecting them. Studies have revealed that nondisclosure of HIV/AIDS promoted the spread of HIV/AIDS.

Findings in this study revealed that women were subjects to men in everything, including sexual encounters. Participants reported their inability to request the use of condom by their husbands during sexual intimacy. Such request was met with punishment from the husband. Though risk perception was high, it did not prevent them from engaging in risky sexual behaviors. The widely held belief was that, when a woman asked for protection such as a condom from the husband, such woman was deemed promiscuous and would be punished through abandonment or divorce.

Findings also revealed that the subservient role of women placed them as subjects to men. According to all the participants, women had to obey their husbands in everything. They had to be willing to have sex anytime he requested it. Though they were in constant fear of HIV/AIDS, their orientation was to always be ready to have sexual intimacy with their husbands so he would love them more and see them as the obedient wife. This brought competition among wives to cut the favor of the husband. It was regarded as a booster to the man's ego when his wives were competing to seek his favor and have sex with him. Competition resulted in using a plan to apportion a day for each wife to sleep with the husband. Not only did this act infringe on the freedom of women, it allowed for extramarital affairs by women who were not satisfied. Although participants did not mention extramarital affairs as one of their coping skills, it appeared to be one. Extramarital affairs in polygamy was a precursor to the spread of HIV/AIDS (Sadiq et al. 2010; Nyathikazi et al. 2013).

# CHAPTER 19

## Social Change Implication

The social change implication is to reduce the prevalence of HIV/AIDS in Nigeria by advocating for safer sex practices among people who are married into polygamy as a cultural belief. It is expected that the information gathered from this interview will help the Nigerian Ministry of Health, the Nigerian Ministry of Education, and other health program developers to develop an initiative, such as the female condom, to empower the Nigerian woman to prevent HIV/AIDS. It is also expected that the information will help the younger generation to make informed decisions when getting married. At the community level, this information will be presented to the community leaders in rural cities of Nigeria, where polygamy is more prevalent. This information will be used to campaign for prevention of HIV/AIDS through safe sex, screened blood transfusion, and non-sharing of needles and syringes. Health workers will make the presentation in form of seminars and community conferences. Health workers will be encouraged to participate in staff training and development programs that enhance their knowledge of HIV/AIDS by using this information.

At the organization level, this information will be useful for mass media organizations to launch campaigns against polygamy without safe sex practices for those who are married into polygamy and to campaign against polygamy for the younger generation. The ultimate goal is to desist from the negative health behavior of polygamy so as to reduce the prevalence of HIV/AIDS.

## Conclusion

This interview confirms that polygamy is a high risk for spreading HIV/AIDS. This presents an opportunity for program developers to create initiatives that prevents HIV/AIDS in the rural communities of Nigeria where polygamy is more prevalent. From these findings, women are at a disadvantage when it comes to preventing sexually transmitted diseases, including HIV/AIDS. Findings also reveal that there is a high level of stigma attached to HIV/AIDS that results in discrimination against HIV-positive individuals. Perhaps this could be attributed to lack of adequate knowledge regarding the transmission of the disease. It is important to create prevention programs that focus on women due to their perceived risk of HIV/AIDS. Community-based programs and mass media organizations should reinforce monogamy as a normative practice. A long-term community-based program will increase knowledge and consequently reduce the stigma attached to HIV/AIDS. It is expected that, with increase in knowledge about HIV/AIDS and awareness of prevention methods, women will be empowered to protect themselves from HIV/AIDS infection.

# CHAPTER 20

I used the health belief model (HBM) to evaluate the perception of the women about HIV/AIDS and their attitude toward the risk that polygamy poses for HIV/AIDS. I submit that this model helps to affirm the findings of the study and will subsequently help in dissemination of findings to stakeholders. The general construct of the HBM model is shown in figure 2.

The HBM is a psychological model that attempts to explain and predict health behaviors. This is done by focusing on the attitudes and beliefs of individuals. Social psychologists Hochbaum, Rosenstock, and Kegels, all working in the US Public Health Services, first developed the HBM in the 1950s. The HBM has four constructs: perceived susceptibility, perceived severity, perceived benefits, and perceived barriers (Sharma 2011).

I used the general construct of the HBM model to better understand and synthesize the findings of the research. This study reveals that there is perceived susceptibility to HIV/AIDS with women interviewed. All admitted that they were at risk of contracting HIV/AIDS when they were practicing polygamy (perceived susceptibility). All admitted that they knew the severity of HIV/AIDS. They knew that polygamy promoted the

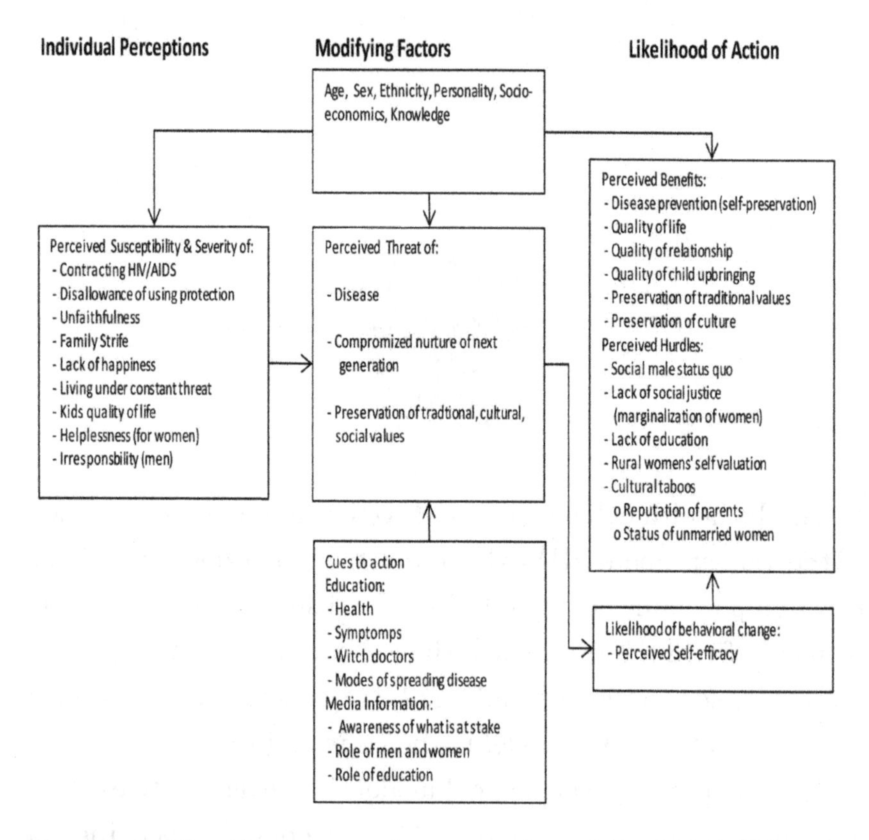


**Figure 2.** The diagrammatic expression of the HBM (Glanz et al. 2002, 52).

spread of HIV/AIDS, but they could not refuse their husbands sex or demand he use protection (perceived severity). They all admitted that they were in constant fear of HIV/AIDS, which indicated that they knew it would be beneficial to be able to prevent the disease (perceived benefits). Those who had a high perception of risk were more likely to seek intervention (Nyathikazi 2013). The barriers mentioned were the responses of their husbands to use of condom, which could be beating, abandonment, or divorce.

In close relationship to the four constructs are cues to action and self-efficacy, which Rosenstock and others added in 1988. Cues to action would activate Nigerian women's readiness to change the risky behavior. Self-efficacy reveals the level of confidence of the women in their ability to change the risky behavior. Changing a risky behavior in this study involves preventing HIV/AIDS for the women who are in polygamy and attempting to stop polygamy by informing the younger generation of its negative consequences.

Critically thinking about all these factors in the perspective of Nigerian rural women's mind-set brings to light a bigger picture that includes many factors that can be influenced to mitigate the negative consequences of polygamy. The problem that the rural Nigerian community is exposed to is seemingly much larger than just HIV. Beyond the obvious threat to individual health, the phenomenon under study appears to be impacting both the sociocultural values and quality of upbringing of the future generations. I have attempted to include the bigger picture of the imminent threat into the perceived threat of the HBM model. The approach of making people realize the higher stakes may help generate momentum required to trigger the sense of efficacy that would be required for the rural Nigerian community to face the challenge. This approach could also enable the local nongovernmental organizations (NGOs) and government organizations to approach the problem from multiple view angles.

As an example, a public appeal to bring about a change can be based on not only medical grounds but also on the grounds of saving rural culture from getting corrupted, securing a brighter future for next generations. A depiction of these ideas is captured in figure 3 below.

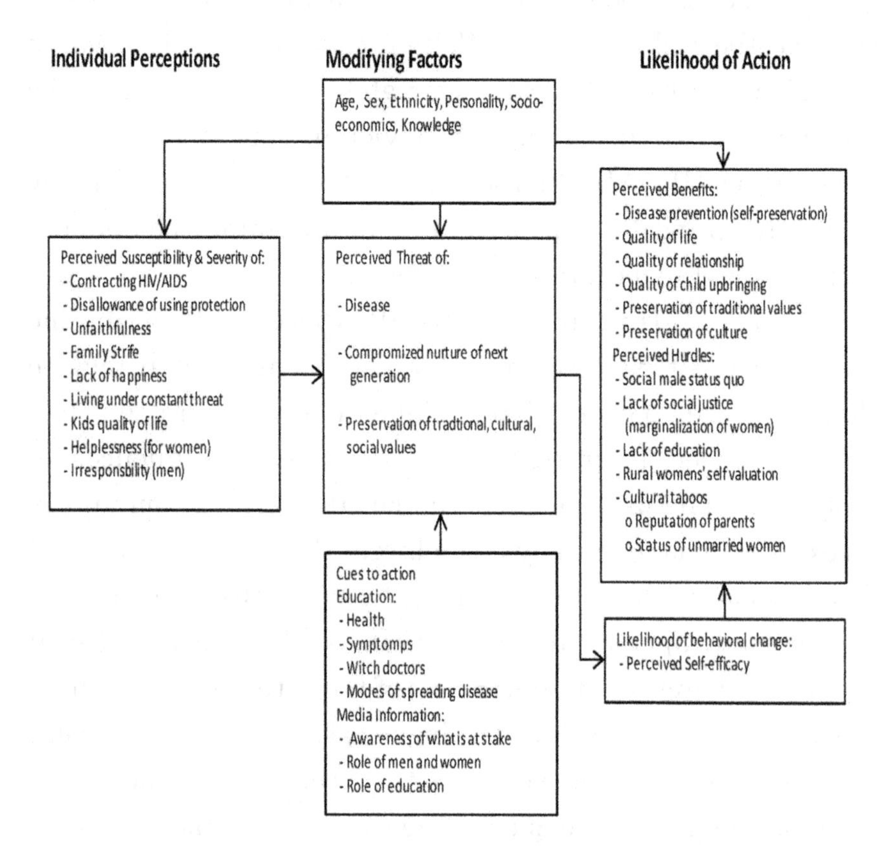


**Figure 3.** Barriers to action.

# INTERVIEW NOTES

## Bearing Witness to Polygamy and the Perception of HIV/AIDS: Lived Experiences

**Name**

P1

**What is your age?**

Forty-two

**How long have you been in America?**

Ten years

**What is your marital status?**

Married

**How long have you been married in America?**

Eight years

**What is your present level of education?**

College

**Probe: How many years of college education do you have and what is your specialty?**

One year. Licensed practical nurse (LPN).

**What is your present occupation?**

LPN

**How old were you when you got married to your husband in Nigeria?**

Eighteen

**How old was your husband in Nigeria when you got married to him?**

Twenty-four

**Was this your first marriage? And how long?**

Yes. Fourteen years.

**Was your marriage arranged?**

No.

**Did you marry for love, family obligation, or another reason?**

No, I didn't marry for love. I married for family obligation. It is important in my family that we marry so as to be a pride of our community and to have children. If we don't marry, we cannot achieve these.

**Probe: So you didn't love your husband when you married him?**

No, if I love him, I will not be able to allow him to marry another wife. We women are brought up to expect that our husband will marry many wives.

**Were you happy knowing that he will marry many wives?**

Yes, because I will have somebody to help me with cooking, cleaning, etc., and when I am pregnant, he will have someone to sleep with.

**How did you feel about getting married?**

I was happy I had a man who wanted me to be his wife, and I was happy that it was time for me to have children.

**Did your family approve of your prospective husband?**

Yes, they liked him.

**Did your mother discuss marriage with multiple wives with you?**

Yes, and she also taught me how to be obedient to my husband and live peacefully with my co-wives. We also learn about multiple wives as we grow up because we are born into it.

**What did your mother tell you?**

She would always say the wife is subject to the husband in everything. She cannot take decisions for him or for herself and the children. She must always be available for sex and treat other wives' children like her own.

**Did your father discuss marriage with multiple wives with you?**

Yes, he was always talking to me about each person's roles in the home.

**Probe: What did he say about roles?**

I saw the roles as I was growing up, and he would also tell me that the man is the authority man in the home. He is the decision maker and provider, and everything in the home belongs to him.

**What was your education status in Nigeria? And did you graduate?**

High school. Yes, I graduated.

**What was the education status of your husband in Nigeria? And did he graduate?**

Teacher training. Yes, he graduated.

**What was your occupation in Nigeria?**

Hairdressing

**Why did you change your occupation to LPN when you relocated here?**

Nursing is more in demand here, and there is good pay.

**How were you able to get the money to go to school here?**

I trained as LNA when I came here and worked to save for LPN. My husband helped pay too.

**What was the occupation of your husband?**

Sixth-grade math teacher

**How many other wives did your husband have? And what were their ages?**

He had three other wives. They were younger than me. The last one was nineteen when he married her.

**How did you feel when each new wife came into the house?**

I always had mixed feelings. Because I expected it, it was not strange to me, but I wished we were not many so as to get my husband's attention. So I was neither happy nor sad.

**What was your position among the wives?**

I was the first.

**As the first, did you make decisions for other wives?**

If it has to do with taking care of our husband or when our husband is not around, yes, but if it has to do with the wives, our husband makes our decisions.

**Probe: Why did your husband make your decisions?**

It is our tradition that the husband makes the decision for his family.

**Probe: So the first wife is the most powerful of the wives.**

Yes, she is supposed to be, but the favorite wife, who is usually the last wife, sometimes takes over because she gets everything like money, gifts, and attention from the husband.

**Were you the favorite?**

No. The last wife was the favorite.

**How did you feel?**

I felt jealous, but I have had my own time too.

**Did she obey your instructions?**

Yes, when our husband is there. When he is not there, she doesn't obey me.

**Did you report her to your husband?**

No, she may tell a lie on me, and our husband would believe her, being the favorite at that time.

**How many children lived in the home?**

I had four children. We don't count other people's children.

**How were resources divided among the children in the home?**

Our husband gives each child money for personal use and school every week according to how much their needs are. They put their needs on a piece of paper and give to him. The younger ones are given equal amounts of money through their mother. He gives the most senior wife money for food every week.

**Where are your children now?**

They are here in U.S.

**How old are they?**

Twenty-three, twenty-one, nineteen, and seventeen

**Do they miss their father?**

No, they rarely talk about him, but they miss their siblings.

**How would you describe your relationship with your husband in Nigeria?**

It was not a good one because there were other wives and many girlfriends. He stopped showing love to me from the time he married the second wife. We did not have love toward each other because you cannot do that in polygamy if you want peace in your home. Some men do it by showing favoritism to the youngest wife. That was what my husband did at a time, and because of that, there were always fights in our home. Other wives will be fighting the new wife out of jealousy.

**Tell me more about not showing love.**

In polygamy, it is a rule that the husband should not show love to a wife more than others except when she is a new wife. That doesn't last long so that others will not be jealous. Some men don't show love at all so that there will be no fight. Women don't show love too so that there will be no jealousy except when they actually want to fight.

**Did your husband tell all of you and the children when a new wife was coming?**

No, he doesn't have to do that. He just brings them, and wives and the children accept them.

**How would you describe the other wives of your husband in Nigeria?**

They were all bitches, always fighting one another. The last one was my husband's favorite. She was just bitchy. She infected my husband with HIV. Both of them are sick now.

**Did you all live together?**

Yes.

**How could you all avoid one another so there would be no fight?**

We can't do that in the same house.

**Tell me about your relationship with other wives.**

Not good at all. We were always fighting.

**Did anyone try to make peace?**

Yes, our children.

**Probe: Did the fight end at one point?**

No, it is an ongoing thing in polygamy. We can pretend that we like one another in the presence of our husband, but at his back, it is fight to finish.

**Probe: Do the children fight too?**

Oh, yes, they side with their mothers during the fight. After the fights, the older ones bring everybody together and make peace.

**How do children get along?**

They play, eat, study, and do everything together. They like one another.

**Probe: Tell me more about the fight. Was it physical or verbal?**

Verbal

**How did you do it verbally?**

We shouted and call each other names.

**Probe: What was your husband doing about it?**

He didn't know about it.

**Probe: What happens if he knows about it?**

He would be mad with us and scold us or slap us, depending on how he feels.

**Probe: Did that ever happen?**

Yes, many times.

**Was the favorite wife scolded or slapped less than others?**

Yes.

**How did that make you feel when you were not the favorite wife?**

I felt very bad and cried in my room. My children would cry with me too without understanding what was happening. They would feel it is the normal thing for Father to beat Mother.

**How would you describe your experience of polygamy?**

It was not good. There was no love. Everything was competition among wives. I was in constant fear of STDs. My husband was too domineering, and we can't question him. It was horrible. If not for the culture, I will not do it. I was not happy at all. I was just taking care of my children.

**What do you mean by the culture?**

It is our belief that a woman should stay married and obey her husband for life.

**What was the competition about?**

To get our husband's attention, they cook him special meals and dress up provocatively.

**Were they getting his attention?**

Yes.

**How were you taking care of your children?**

I spent all the money he gave the children on them instead of using some to buy dresses for myself to compete like they [co-wives] were doing.

**Probe: Why did you stay married to him when you were not happy?**

I had to have a husband to have children. If I don't have a husband, my family will not be proud of me, and I will be seen as a prostitute in the community.

**Probe: You said you were a hairdresser. That means you were working, right?**

Yes.

**Probe: Who provides the money for living expenses?**

The husband has to provide. That is what makes him a real man.

**Probe: What if he doesn't provide? Would you be the one to provide?**

If he doesn't provide, I will provide for myself and my children.

**Would that be a shame on him?**

Yes, he cannot command anymore. No man likes that so they don't allow it to happen.

**Probe: Can you leave him if he doesn't provide for the family?**

If I leave, he will not release my children. I can't leave my children with a man who will not take care of them and with wives who were always fighting. What is my essence in life if my children are suffering?

**Can you sue him for custody?**

No, that doesn't happen where I lived. The man owns the children.

**If you leave, where would you go?**

I don't have anywhere to go. My parents will send me back. Once you marry, you belong to the husband.

**How did you cope?**

I was just keeping to myself. It was the culture. So I could not do anything. I was just hoping day after day that all will be well.

**What was the role of your husband in polygamy?**

He was the breadwinner and the head of the family. He was also the decision maker, and we had to obey him whether his decision is good or bad.

**Give me an example of a bad decision that he made.**

He always teaches his children how to smoke and drink, and no wife can stop him. When I tried to advise him against it, he slapped and kicked me.

**What did you do to make your children not follow the example?**

Nothing. I had no power to do anything. If the children don't do as he taught them, he will know I was responsible, and that is trouble for me.

**Please tell me what you knew then about HIV/AIDS.**

It is a killer disease. That's the way they describe it. It is transmitted through sex, and once you get it, you are dead. Knowing this, we started fighting the prostitutes because of our husbands. Nobody in the village would have anything to do with you if you have HIV, except your family members. In the hospitals in the city, they treated them separately. The village hospitals don't accept them so they turned to traditional healers. The people started to hide it, and many people were infected and died. I was one of those people who did not take HIV/AIDS seriously until I saw people very sick and die of it. People were dying so much of HIV/AIDS that it became a song in the village where I lived.

**What kind of song?**

The radio people were singing the song in their adverts to describe HIV/AIDS.

**Probe: How did you know it is a killer disease?**

Through TV and radio.

**Did the traditional medicine cure them?**

No.

**What happens when they are not cured?**

They stay with the healer because it is cheaper. I believe it is only HIV/AIDS that they can't cure. They cure other disease so the people trust the herbs.

**Probe: Tell me more about fighting the prostitutes. How did you fight them?**

We always warn them against our husbands. If they don't stop, we fight them physically with the help of young street boys.

**Probe: How about telling your husband to stop going to prostitutes?**

No, we can't do that. No wife can do that. We fear our husbands too much to do that.

**Probe: Why?**

Because it can result in anything like beating or any kind of punishment.

**Probe: If he beats you, what action can you take against him?**

Nothing. We cannot even talk about it. The wife will be seen as a bad wife. What happens in your family stays in your family.

**How did you feel about that?**

I feel bad, but there is nothing we can do.

**Probe: What if you get sick from the beating?**

We take care of ourselves

**Probe: You don't go to the hospital?**

No.

**Probe: Why?**

It is a constant thing so the body gets used to it, and it is not a huge beating that can land me in hospital. It is something like two or three slaps or five strokes of cane. We only go to hospital if it is much.

**What would be much?**

Like if I have injury.

**Probe: Who pays for the hospital bills when you go?**

If he likes, he pays. If he doesn't pay, we pay. That's why I don't go.

**Can you go to hospital for other ailments?**

Yes, if I have the money. If I don't, I will go to traditional healer.

**What is your opinion about polygamy and HIV/AIDS?**

Polygamy is one of the ways by which HIV/AIDS spreads in Nigeria. Somebody catches it, and everybody is infected. Even if you are sure about yourself, how about the other wives? Our husband can get it from anybody and infect us. You know men are polygamous by nature. If men can just keep to one wife, there will be no HIV/AIDS.

**Probe: You mentioned other wives. If they have HIV, would they not disclose it?**

Nobody discloses it. If they disclose it, they are sent out. Where would they say they got it? Not from our husband because men don't admit they have disease. They cannot talk about having extramarital affairs, though some wives have secret boyfriends in the community that they buy gifts for so as to keep the affairs secret.

**What happens when the man gets really sick?**

We will take him to the traditional healer.

**How do they get the boys in the community?**

They approach the young boys with gifts and ask them to be their boyfriends.

**What kind of gifts?**

It is usually money.

**How do they get the money if they are not working?**

They save it up from food money or borrow from friends.

**How do they meet the boys?**

They start with flirting with the boys, and later they give them money.

**How long does it last?**

Till the boy gets married.

**How does this affair make the wife feel?**

They feel good about it. It satisfies their sexual urges that their husband doesn't have time to satisfy.

**How did you perceive your risk for HIV/AIDS when you were in polygamy?**

I knew I was at risk, but what can I do in a system where the wife cannot talk? We are not treated as equals, so we cannot make decisions about anything, including sex, so we are at risk of anything. If I complain, he will abandon me or send me out. It is the system. It is not possible to stop the men. If anyone tries that, they are just promoting extramarital affairs. The women know that men cannot satisfy all the wives, so some women look outside the marriage for satisfaction and therefore infect the husband who, in turn, infects others. I was just hoping that I would not get it. I knew I was at risk, but women are usually faithful in marriage because it is against the culture for a married woman to be seen with another man, but the man is the one who brings HIV by sleeping with different women. There must have been a sexual relationship between them before he decides to marry her. Men are polygamous by nature. There are many examples in the Bible, even though God made one man and one woman. Trust me. Polygamists go about sampling women in bed before marrying the most sexually active one. By so doing, they acquire and spread HIV.

**Do the men go out to have an affair to spite the woman?**

Yes.

**Probe: You said some women go outside the marriage for sex, but you also said women are usually faithful. Please explain further.**

Yes, women are trained to be faithful, but if the man cannot satisfy them, they go out secretly to have a boyfriend, usually a younger man, for sex. Most women don't do it, because of the curse attached to it.

**Probe: A curse? Can you tell me more about that?**

It is a cultural belief that women who go outside their marriage for sex die young.

**Probe: Have you ever seen one die young?**

No, but that is because not many women do it.

**Probe: You mentioned that he will send you out if you complain. Where would you go? And what happens to your children?**

I will have to go back to my parents or family members if they will accept me. As for children, men don't allow women to take their children except if they are too young. So I will have to leave them behind. No woman wants to do that, and that's why we stay.

**How did you get them here with you?**

My children were old enough when I was coming here. I did not bring them all at once. When my brother invited me here, I came with the two youngest and arranged for the remaining.

**Did the ones you left stay with your husband?**

Yes, but my mother was nearby and was checking on them.

**Was your husband willing to release the ones you brought?**

Yes, it is a thing of pride to men when their children are abroad.

**Probe: I am curious why your husband allowed you to join your brother here, knowing it is shame to a woman to leave her husband.**

My brother knows the culture is wrong, so he took me away from it as soon as he could do it.

**Has he helped your other siblings?**

Yes, he is helping as many as he can help.

**How did your knowledge of HIV/AIDS affect your sexual relationship with your husband when you were in polygamy?**

I was always afraid to the point of crying when it was my turn for sex because I know I was open to infection since he has other women, but I have to do it according to the plan. No protection. Nothing. No woman can ask for that. Except if you are ready for false accusation and divorce from the husband, you cannot demand protection. If I ask for condom, he will suspect me of using it with a boyfriend and divorce me. No woman wants to live alone in a society where divorced women are treated like prostitutes. I was just taking antibiotics, but I was doing it secretly so that he will not send me out or accuse me of not trusting him.

**If the husband knows about extramarital affairs, what would he do to the boy?**

Nothing. He will only punish his wife.

**Probe: Who prescribed antibiotics for HIV for you?**

Nobody, but I knew people use it for infection.

**How did you know?**

I have friends who were getting it from the hospital

**How?**

Through their friends.

**Do you think it worked?**

No. I am a nurse now. I know antibiotics do not work for viruses. At that time, I thought it worked.

**You talked about sleeping with your husband according to plan. What plan?**

That is a roster for who sleeps with the husband at a particular day in the week. It is like apportioning a day for a wife to sleep with him. We all know our days, and we don't take another woman's day except when she is pregnant or menstruating.

**How is your relationship with your husband in your present marriage where you do not practice polygamy?**

We are very much in love. We respect each other. We married for love and have a child together. We decide together. He is Nigerian and had a child from his previous marriage in Nigeria. He was not polygamous. His wife refused to come here with him when he came here eighteen years ago. His wife had since remarried and sent the child to him. We all live together in harmony.

**Did you grow up in a city or rural village?**

Rural village. We have a mix of educated and uneducated people. Many of the older people were businesspeople. The younger ones were a mix of civil servants and businesspeople.

**If you had grown up in a city, do you believe the issue of marriages with multiple wives would be accepted?**

Yes, polygamy is accepted in the city too, but it is more common in the rural regions.

**Why is it more common in the rural regions?**

Because we are not as educated as the city people, so we don't have anything we are doing after primary or high school. Unless people go to the city for higher education, they get into business. Men begin to learn a trade from primary school, and women are being prepared for marriage after primary school.

**Looking back to that system, what do you feel about the idea of being prepared for marriage after primary school?**

I don't like it at all. It doesn't allow the woman to mature.

**Did the multiple wives live in the same house?**

Yes, all of us live together with our husband and children.

**What kind of struggles were there in day-to-day living arrangements with multiple wives and children?**

We all had our different rooms. Each wife and her children live in one room separate from the husband. We all share same living room and eat together. In our house, we had two bathrooms and one kitchen. The only struggle we have with the bathrooms is, when both are occupied and someone needs to go out urgently, he will have to wait and call on the person inside the bathroom to be quick. Anyone who didn't want to be delayed will have to wake up earlier than other people to use the bathroom. Children of multiple wives get along or quarrel depending on the rules of the house and how properly the husband handles the affairs of the home. In my home, our children were good with one another until we, their mothers, start to fight. They take sides, but after the fight, they make peace with one another first and come together to settle their mothers.

**Can you describe your cultural traditions about marriage in some detail?**

Our cultural traditions about marriage involve a man finding a woman, talking to her, or going through her parents to talk to her. Sometimes the discussion goes from parents to parents. A parent likes a girl or boy, talks to the parents of the girl or boy, and exchanges gifts. The boy marries the girl after paying the bride price, and she becomes his wife forever. No room for divorce except if she has extramarital affairs. The man can divorce the wife, but the woman cannot divorce the man. If she is divorced, no man will marry her. The man provides for the whole family and makes decisions for everybody. He can marry as many wives as he wants without telling his wife and children ahead. Some men tell their wives to choose their next wives. In marriage, the families of both husband and wife become one family and give gifts to each other. The children of the marriage belong to the husband, especially the male child. If the man divorces his wife, the wife cannot go with the children, except if they are too young or old enough to make decisions for themselves as to who they want to stay with.

**What is the youngest a woman gets married?**

In my village, the youngest is sixteen because that is when we get out of school for those of us who go to school.

**Can women remain unmarried into their twenties or thirties if they wish to get advanced education and a career?**

Yes, but such women don't stay in the village because no man will want to marry them. They will be too civilized for the husband to handle. Except if they get a man who has advanced education like themselves, which is rare in the village, such women will stay unmarried for their lives, and that cannot happen in the village. They will be labelled as prostitutes, and other women will be fighting them away from their husbands. It will be a shame to their parents.

**Do you believe you would have left your village to marry outside if you had gone beyond high school?**

Yes, I would have left, and I wouldn't have married the man I married because he wouldn't have measured up to my standard at all. Most university-educated people don't practice polygamy.

**Do you regret not going to the university?**

Yes, I do, and that is why, when I got the opportunity here to go to college, I used it.

**Would you ever count the children from other wives as part of your extended family on any level?**

No, we don't count other people's children.

**Why not?**

We believe it is a sin to count people's children. I think the people got that belief from the Bible where King David counted the Israelites and the people died. I have never asked why.

**If one of those other children called you now for help, do you believe you would help him or her?**

Yes, we treat co-wives' children as ours. If they need my help, I will surely help them.

**How did your children feel about being part of that extended family with other wives and children when you were in Nigeria?**

When they were young, my children liked the idea of having many children that they can play with in the house. As they grew up, they started to question why they have so many mothers [wives are called mothers] and siblings. It is when they start to ask questions like that that we start to teach them about our beliefs regarding multiple wives and large families.

**Do your adult children ever talk about that part of their lives now? How do they describe their feelings?**

Yes, they talk about it.They hate it now.

**Do your children feel any influence of Nigerian cultural traditions on their relationships in the United States?**

No, they have forgotten almost all the cultural beliefs because we don't teach them here. Their relationships are with their schoolmates here. The boys don't treat their girls like slaves, and the girls don't fear their boyfriends like I did with their father. They are also free to express themselves, and they are happy they are not thinking of polygamy at all in their marriage.

**Do you feel any influence of Nigerian cultural traditions on your relationships with men in the U.S.?**

No. Nigerian men get here and become civilized. They don't practice what they practice at home here. Some of them who treat their wives here like they do in Nigerian pay dearly for it because their wives call the cops on them and they end up in jail. I think, because they are more civilized and don't want trouble, they treat their wives with respect here. My present husband is Nigerian, and he treats me with respect.

**Would you provide encouragement to your daughter if she wishes to move back to Nigeria and have a traditional marriage?**

No, I will never do that. That type of marriage is nothing to be proud of.

**Could a wife in a traditional marriage in Nigeria with multiple wives ever refuse sex with her husband?**

No, never. She has to allow him any time any day. If she would refuse, she must have a strong reason like menstruating or pregnancy. No other reason, not even sickness or tiredness. If she refuses, the husband will be suspecting her of extramarital affairs, which is enough ground to divorce her.

**When wives are divorced, do they go back to their parents?**

Yes, and it becomes a shame to their parents.

**What happens to the children?**

As for children, men don't allow women to take their children except if they are too young. So I will have to leave them behind. No woman wants to do that, and that's why we stay.

**What did wives of one husband typically fight about?**

When they are jealous that the wife is receiving too much attention from the husband, like if she is seen with him all the time. Sometimes they tell lies about one another to shift their husband's attention from the one they are accusing. Sometimes it is about their children getting less money from the husband than the other. That happens at times if the needs of one child is greater than the other, and the husband has to give more to the child with the greater need.

**When you were slapped or caned by your husband, was there anyone you could ever go to for support? For example, a friend or mother?**

No, we don't talk to anyone about it. What happens in our home stays in our home. If we tell anyone, they will call us bad wives.

**Were there any laws that support a wife who was hurt by her husband? For example, could she ever call the police for support if severely beaten? In any of the large cities, were there any women's groups that support wives?**

In the village, there is no such thing. If there is injury, we treat it ourselves. In the city, they can go to elders to settle between husband and wife. The elders will call them together and make peace. Usually they tell the wife to listen to her husband. If there is a need to call the cops, it would be that the wife died from the beating. When that happens, the man will be charged to court. In the village, if the wife dies from the husband's beatings, she will be buried by the husband and pay to the parents.

**Probe: Is that like paying back the bride price?**

He will pay double the bride price because he killed her.

**Do you know if there is any current movement to change the cultural tradition of multiple wives?**

Yes, in the city, but in the village, I have not heard of any.

**Please talk a little more about the use of traditional healers in villages versus Western medicine doctors. Do women typically use a traditional healer or Western medicine doctors for pregnancy and childbirth?**

Traditional healers are men who are well known in the village as herbalists. They deal in herbs to cure diseases, and some of them make claims of curing all diseases. People in the village go to them more than they go to the hospital because hospital is more expensive. Many people claim the herbs work for them, and yes, we use them when we are pregnant and for delivery.

**What do you think about it?**

I think it works. I have used them during my pregnancies and deliveries.

**What do you think are the benefits of going to a traditional healer versus Western medicine?**

I think the benefits are we trust the herbs and we don't pay much. That is enough to put our mind at rest and heal us. I believe the body heals itself when we can trust that we are putting our health in the hands of people that we trust, unlike Western medicine that we don't know how they made.

**Do you still hold that belief?**

Not anymore. I go to hospital here because I work in the hospital, but if I go home, I will use the herbs.

**Please discuss your faith traditions in Nigeria. For example, what do priests and pastors say about men having multiple wives?**

In the village, they don't condemn it because they too have multiple wives. In the city, they condemn it.

**Could a wife in Nigeria go to a priest or pastor for emotional support in dealing with a husband who has multiple wives and girlfriends?**

Yes, a wife can go to them. They usually ask them to be obedient wives and pray that God should touch the heart of their husbands so that he will love them all.

**Could a woman in Nigeria choose college and career over marriage and be accepted?**

Yes, in the city, not in the village.

**Are girls in Nigeria encouraged to go onto vocational training or university?**

Yes, in the city, not in the village.

# INTERVIEW NOTE

**Name**

P2

**What is your age?**

Forty

**How long have you been in America?**

Nine years

**What is your marital status?**

Married

**How long have you been married in America?**

Six years

**What is your present level of education?**

College

**Probe: How many years of college education do you have, and what is your specialty?**

One year. Licensed practical nurse (LPN)

**Did you graduate?**

Yes.

**What is your present occupation?**

LPN

**What was your education status in Nigeria?**

High school

**What was the education status of your husband in Nigeria?**

None.

**Probe: Do you know why he did not go to school?**

He said he did not like school.

**How old were you when you got married to your husband in Nigeria?**

Eighteen

**How old was your husband in Nigeria when you got married to him?**

Thirty-five

**Was this your first marriage? And how long?**

Yes. Thirteen years.

**How did both of you meet?**

We met in the market where he was selling beef. He was in charge of all the market for beef in our village. We were always going to his stalls to buy beef. One day when I went there to buy beef, he told me that he wanted me to be his wife. After that, we dated for six months and got married.

**How were you dating?**

We were going out to places.

**So it was your choice to marry him?**

Yes.

**Why did you marry him despite the age difference?**

He was very nice to me at that time. He was buying me gifts and taking me out to parties in the city. I enjoyed the attention.

**Did he pay dowries to your parents when he married you?**

Yes, he brought money, yams, drinks, clothing, and so on.

**What was your occupation in Nigeria?**

Housewife

**Why did you do nursing when you relocated to U.S.?**

The jobs are available in nursing, and the pay is good. Besides I decided not to be a housewife here when I have the opportunity to go to college. It was lack of money that made me not to go further than high school in Nigeria.

**How did you get the money to go to college here?**

I worked as a housekeeper in a hotel first and saved money to go to school for nursing assistant (LNA). Then I saved money to go to nursing school, where I did LPN for one year.

**What other occupation did your husband in Nigeria have apart from beef selling?**

None. He made a lot of money from that business.

**How many other wives did your husband have, and what was their ages?**

Six other wives. I don't know their ages.

**Did you all live in the same house?**

Yes.

**What was your position among the wives?**

I was the third wife.

**Do you think he married you because he wanted to have more wives?**

Yes, Nigerian men usually want to marry more wives. It shows that they have money and power to control many women.

**Probe: Who among the wives was giving instructions?**

We do things in order of seniority when it is women's affairs, like cooking, cleaning, shopping for the whole house, etc., but major decisions are made by our husband.

**Probe: What kind of major decisions?**

The major one is about how we spend money.

**Probe: How was he making that decision?**

He would pay our children's school fees. He would give money to each one of us and our children every week for our personal use. He would also put money on our dining table for food for the week. The first wife will then take the money, and all of us will decide what we need in the house and go to the market to buy them. Usually the last wife and older female children cook for the house, but the first wife cooks for our husband. That is the culture.

**What do you mean by culture?**

That is the way we do things in our house.

**Probe: Is this something that has to take that order? Or can you reverse it and be the one to provide money for the whole house?**

No. The man will lose his pride. Our belief is that a man must provide money for his family. If the wife provides for him, he is not a real man and shouldn't have wives. My father provided money for my mother and his other wives too. That is what our men do.

**Did your mother discuss marriages with multiple wives with you?**

Yes.

**Probe: What did your mother tell you?**

She said the husband is superior to the wives. She said there will always be many wives. The wives cannot take decisions for the husband or for herself and the children. She must always be available for sex and treat other wives' children like her own.

**Did your father discuss marriages with multiple wives with you?**

Yes, he was always talking about roles in the home.

**Probe: What did he say about roles?**

He would always tell me that the man is the authority man in the home. He is the decision maker and provider, and everything in the home belongs to him.

**Probe: So you being the third wife among seven wives received and gave instructions?**

Yes. Sometimes the favorite wife gets more powerful than others.

**Probe: So there is a favorite wife?**

Not all the time, but when we have one, we usually know through the attitude of our husband toward a particular wife.

**Probe: What would your husband do to his favorite wife?**

He would give her gifts more than others. He will take her out more and speak well of her. This is not supposed to happen in polygamy, but some men do it.

**Did it happen in your marriage?**

Yes, when I was the last wife, I was the favorite.

**How did it make you feel?**

I felt powerful. I was happy about it, but it didn't last long because he married another wife two years after me, and that one became the favorite.

**Probe: So each time a new wife came, she became the favorite?**

Yes, usually. But that can also change. The second wife of our husband became the favorite at a time when her father became a chief in our village. That was a boost to our husband's ego because he went about boasting about it.

**How did you feel when the second wife became the favorite?**

I was unhappy because I felt she has enjoyed her own time. Then she was having double enjoyment, and our husband did not play it well at all. He would always go out with her and talk about her and her father everywhere. That made the rest of us jealous, but we couldn't do anything, so we just accepted it.

**Were any of the wives working?**

No, we were housewives. Our husband never allowed us to work so that he could control us.

**How many children lived in the home?**

There were many children. More than twenty. Mine was four.

**Where are your children now?**

One is in U.K. Others are here with me.

**How old are they?**

Twenty-one, nineteen, seventeen, and sixteen

**If you had grown up in a city, do you believe the issue of marriages with multiple wives would be accepted?**

Yes, polygamy is accepted in the city too, but it is more common in the rural regions.

**Why is it more common in the rural regions?**

Because we are not as educated as the city people, so we don't have anything we are doing after primary or high school. Unless people go to the city for higher education, they get into business. Men begin to learn a trade from primary school, and women are being prepared for marriage after primary school.

**How would you describe your relationship with your husband in Nigeria?**

It was just the custom to be married. If not, there is nothing about the relationship. I had to obey him in everything. I could not make any decision. He would shut me up. I was afraid of him. Anything he says about me is what the people will accept. He was making my decisions for me because women have no voice in our culture.

**What do you mean it was the custom to be married?**

Marriage is something that is compulsory in Nigeria. If you are not married and you have children, your children are regarded as bastards, and your family will not be proud of you because people will blame them for not bringing you up properly. So when you are married, you are a pride to your family. And if the husband is rich, it is double blessing.

**How is it double blessing?**

My husband was giving money to my family whenever they visited.

**Tell me more about what you mean by anything he says about you is what people will believe.**

People believe whatever a man says about his wife. If he says I am a good wife, people will believe him. If he says I am bad, they will also believe him. There is no respect for women at all.

**What do you think he should have done to show you respect?**

He should give me a chance to talk and listen to me, but no, that doesn't happen at all. If a Nigerian man does that, his friends and family will not regard him as a real man.

**Probe: So in Nigeria, a real man is the one who has many wives and controls them, feeds them, and talks for them.**

Yes.

**How would you describe the other wives of your husband in Nigeria?**

They are nothing to write home about at all. Always fighting and doing wicked things to people. Very jealous and manipulative.

**When they fight, what do they do?**

They beat each other up and call each other all sorts of names.

**Were you involved in the fights?**

Yes, once in a while.

**What was causing the fights?**

Anything from children to husband to food, just anything.

**Did people come to separate you when you fight?**

Yes, our children and the people around.

**Probe: So you did not see eye-to-eye at all when you were living together.**

Not at all.

**Probe: Did the children fight too?**

Yes, when the wives fight, the children side with their mothers and call the wives names.

**Probe: Was it physical?**

No, usually verbal.

**How do the children get along?**

They play together until wives start to fight, and even after the fight, they quickly reconcile and settle the quarrels among wives. The children always want to live peacefully together unlike other wives. Our children go to same schools and eat and study together.

**Tell me about your relationship with other wives.**

We were not on good terms, but we pretend when our husband is around.

**Probe: If your husband knew you were fighting, what would he do?**

He will scold us in the presence of all the people. Or slap and kick us.

**Probe: What would the people do?**

Nothing. We are his wife. He can do whatever he likes with us.

**When he beats you, do you go to the hospital for treatment?**

No, it is not something we take to hospital.

**Probe: Don't you get injured from the beating at all?**

If we get injured, we go to hospital.

**Who pays the hospital bill?**

If he likes, he pays. If he doesn't like, I will have to pay. If I don't have money, I will ask my family members. That is why we don't really go to hospital for things like that.

**How would you describe your experience of polygamy?**

It was not good at all. Everybody suspects everybody. There was no love.

**Probe: Between husband and wife?**

Yes, the love is just for the time the wife is new. As soon as she starts having children or another wife comes, the love is over. There was STDs around. I was always afraid. I could not complain if I have an infection. He will suspect me and not himself. He will beat me up in public and send me out of his house. It was a terrible experience. If he likes, he can show love to one wife in the presence of other wives. He can punish his wives publicly. He will be seen as a real man.

**How do you know there was STDs around?**

I had an infection once, and I had to tell my friend who worked at the hospital. She gave me antibiotics.

**Did it work?**

Yes, and I was taking it anytime I felt like I was going to have an infection.

**Probe: You mentioned that he will send you out if you complain. Where would you go? And what happens to your children?**

I will go back to my father's house, of course, and the children will stay with him. You see why we don't leave? We need to stay and take care of our children.

**Probe: When he beats you up in public, do people come to your rescue?**

Yes.

**Probe: What happens when people come to your rescue?**

They just separate us and tell me to be obedient to him.

**Probe: Is there no one to report him to? Like an elder in the community or a social organization for women?**

What? Our society frowns against that. If you report your husband or talk about him badly, you are seen as a bad wife who can destroy the husband. We have to keep everything to ourselves.

**What would the society do to you if you report him? Is there a punishment to that?**

No, but they will just label you as a bad wife.

**How did you cope living in polygamy?**

I was praying and watching. Anytime I suspected anything, I would play sick so that he won't touch me, but that can only last a few days. I was also watching not to annoy our husband. I have seen a wife die from beating. I don't want my children to become motherless.

**Anytime you suspect anything like what?**

STDs.

**Probe: When the wife died from beating, what did her family do?**

Her family met with the man and talked to him over it. He apologized, and that was it. She was his wife. There is little her family could do.

**Who was responsible for the burial?**

The husband, of course.

**What happened to her children after her death?**

Her two children grew up with their evil father and wicked wives. They were not cared for at all. They dropped out of school and were roaming about the streets. Sometimes they would go to their late mother's family for food.

**Why didn't the late mother's family send them to school?**

They didn't have money.

**What was the role of your husband in polygamy?**

He was the breadwinner, and he was doing that very well. He always boasted that he is a superman because he was feeding many people in his house.

**Probe: So everybody depended on him for providing money for the home.**

Yes.

**Probe: If he doesn't provide, can you or other wives provide?**

If I had the money, I will provide if he doesn't provide, but we were all housewives so we don't have money. Some men deliberately make their wives housewives so as to be able to control them.

**Probe: Tell me more about that controlling.**

Because we all depend on him for a living, we have to obey him.

**Please tell me what you knew then about HIV/AIDS.**

We were told that the disease is a killer disease.

**Probe: By whom?**

Radio and TV.

**Probe: Was it through advertisement?**

Yes, and through drama and song. Once they get it, they have a few more years to live, and people will treat them like an outcast.

**How do people treat them like outcasts?**

Nobody would eat, play, or work with them, except their family members and their traditional healers that they go to when the hospitals reject them. People were getting it through sex and were dying everywhere. When my friend had the first child, she was fine, but the second child was a different story. The child started feeling sick all the time. They thought it was sickle cell. When they took him to the hospital, they discovered he had HIV. Then they tested all other members of the family and discovered that it was only the first child that was negative. The husband was a bus driver who was going on tour for days. Who knows which of them had been having extramarital affairs?

**Probe: When the hospital workers discovered that they had HIV, did they take care of them?**

No, they sent them home and advised them to eat well and rest. The people turned to traditional healers.

**Who are traditional healers?**

They are herbalists in the community. People usually go to them instead of hospitals.

**Why do people prefer them to hospitals?**

Because they don't charge much and they are well-known and respected.

**What is your opinion about the traditional medicines?**

They don't work. The people eventually die.

**What is your opinion about polygamy and HIV/AIDS?**

Polygamy is responsible for the amount of HIV/AIDS in Nigeria and Africa in general. The men keep infecting their wives in the name of culture. Take away polygamy, and see if HIV/AIDS will not reduce.

**Probe: How do you think it can be taken away?**

By talking to the young men to marry one wife. And the young women not to marry a married man. Show them examples of people who died of HIV/AIDS. Maybe they will listen.

**Looking back to that system, what do you feel about the idea of being prepared for marriage after primary school?**

I don't like it at all. It doesn't allow the woman to mature.

**How did you perceive your risk for HIV/AIDS when you were in polygamy?**

I was at high risk. Imagine a man trying to satisfy many women sexually. Many of the wives go outside for satisfaction and bring HIV with them. The husband will have sex with her and transfer it to other wives. All of us were at risk, but girls are brought up to know that, in our culture, our men will surely marry many wives because that is the nature of men so I was prepared for it. I know I was at risk of HIV/AIDS, but my children were girls. A female child is not regarded as anybody so I needed to have a male child. If not, he will send me and my daughters out of his house. I had to keep on with the marriage until I had a male child.

**When some wives go outside the home for sex, how does the husband feel?**

He must never know about it.

**Did that happen with you?**

Never.

**How did the women find men outside their marriage?**

They were giving young boys money, and both of them will keep it secret.

**Is it something that goes on for a long time?**

No, it stops when the boy gets married, and they will look for another one.

**If you know about it, can you report the wife to your husband?**

No, they will pay me back terribly. They can plan for me and rope me into something.

**Did you eventually have a male child?**

No.

**What happened when you didn't have a male child?**

He looked for an excuse and sent me out with my daughters, but God helped me through my friend here in the U.S. Now he is claiming his children because they are now doing well.

**How is he claiming them?**

At first, he was sending threats to us through people who come here. Now he is begging his children to come home and bring him here. The children don't answer him.

**Probe: So if the children are all females, the man would send them out.**

Yes. Most times men don't let the children leave until they are old enough to decide. If they are too young, he can let them go with the wife, but if they are all girls, he can send them out if he wants.

**Probe: Can you fight custody in court if he doesn't allow you to go with the male child?**

No. We don't do that.

**How did your knowledge of HIV/AIDS affect your sexual relationship with your husband when you were in polygamy?**

It did not affect it because I had to have children and we must obey him. I was just praying, but I was always afraid. There was this plan that we observe for sex. Sometimes we had a mix-up, and the wives would fight the whole day. The husband sometimes creates the mix-up so as to sleep with the favorite wife. That is the reason men have many wives. If a wife is pregnant or nursing her child, instead of using protection or going outside the marriage, he can satisfy himself with another wife.

**Probe: Tell me more about the plan.**

It is a roster about who sleeps with the husband when. A day is apportioned for each wife to sleep in the husband's room at night.

**Probe: Does it include all wives?**

No, those who are pregnant or nursing are not included.

**How is your relationship with your husband in your present marriage where you do not practice polygamy?**

Very good. We love each other and talk to each other as we like.

**Tell me about your present husband.**

He is Nigerian. He came here when he was twenty years old. He is forty now and has two children with his late wife. I have a child with him. He is a teacher. He allows me to make my decisions, and he is never controlling. We spend money together. We raise our children together and go to places together. My children love him as their own father. He means everything to me.

# INTERVIEW NOTE

**Name**

P3

**What is your age?**

Thirty-nine

**How long have you been in America?**

Six years

**What is your marital status?**

Married

**How long have you been married in America?**

Five years

**What is your present level of education?**

College

**How many years of college? And did you graduate?**

One year. Yes, I graduated.

**What is your present occupation?**

LPN (licensed practical nurse)

**How old were you when you got married to your husband in Nigeria?**

Twenty-one

**How old was your husband in Nigeria when you got married to him?**

Twenty-seven

**Was this your first marriage? And how long?**

No. Twelve years.

**What was your education status in Nigeria?**

High school

**What was the education status of your husband in Nigeria?**

High school

**What was your occupation in Nigeria?**

Trading

**What kind of trade?**

Tailoring and selling clothes

**What was the occupation of your husband?**

Trading

**What kind?**

Selling motor spare parts

**How many other wives did your husband have, and what were their ages?**

He had two other wives. I don't know their ages.

**Were you living in the same house?**

Yes, all of us.

**What was your position among the wives?**

Second wife

**Were you taking instructions from the first wife?**

When I newly came, I was doing that, but not for long. It also depends on the kind of instruction. If it has to do with house chores and women affairs, yes, I would go to her as the first wife. All other decisions were made by our husband.

**What women affairs?**

Cooking and buying foodstuff for the house.

**Probe: Why was your husband making decisions for you?**

That is the culture. If he has a favorite wife among us, she can give instructions too, but it always results in a fight.

**What do you mean the culture?**

That is the normal thing for us. The man is the decision maker of the home. He decides for us and the children on money, school, everything.

**Is that the way of life that you all believe in?**

Yes, and we have to follow it as handed down to us. If a man cannot control his wives, he is not a real man.

**How did you feel about that?**

I felt good about it at that time, but now it is different. My present husband doesn't control me.

**How many children lived in the home?**

Mine was three. We don't count for others.

**Where are your children?**

Here with me in U.S.

**How would you describe your relationship with your husband in Nigeria?**

I don't even know what to call it. Anyway, he was the father of my children. I was the second wife. At first it was good. Later he started sleeping outside. When I asked my senior wife, she said he was like that. I confronted him, and he shouted at me and slapped me. Since then, things were not really good between us because I saw that he deceived me into the marriage.

**Probe: When he slapped you, what did you do?**

Nothing. I can't slap him back.

**Can you report him to somebody among his family or in the community?**

No, that is not acceptable at all. If you talk bad about your husband, you are a bad wife. There is a saying that what happens in the home stays in the home.

**How did you feel about him slapping you?**

I felt unhappy.

**How would you describe the other wives of your husband in Nigeria?**

They are just not good, but we pretended that all was well. Very jealous women.

**Probe: When they showed jealousy, were they fighting physically?**

No, it was more of action and verbal abuse. We were always fighting each other. There was no peace in the house.

**Probe: When you fought, what was your husband's reaction?**

Sometimes he would order us to keep quiet; other times he would leave the house for us and come back later.

**Probe: When he leaves, where does he go to?**

To friends or mistresses. That's why we don't fight in his presence. We don't want him to go out.

**How did you feel each time he left the house like this?**

I fear getting infected because he can go to his mistress, get infected, and bring disease home.

**Tell me about your relationship with other wives.**

Not so good. We fought. We compete.

**How did you compete?**

I buy clothes, shoes, and jewelries for myself and our husband. They are usually same design so that he can wear it when I wear my own. Other wives do it too. We cook special dishes for him too to court his favor.

**What was the favor?**

Taking us out and speaking well about us among his friends.

**Does the fight ever stop?**

No, the fight never stops. It happens all the time.

**Does it involve your children?**

Yes, children side with their mothers and settle them.

**Do they make peace with wives after siding with their mother?**

Yes, the older ones bring the fighting wives together and make peace, and for that period, we will be at peace.

**How would you describe your experience of polygamy?**

It was not good at all. Competition, lies, accusations, fear, etc. Our husband can't show love to anybody so that there will not be fight. We had plans for everything, including sex. I cannot have sex or even play with my husband anytime I like without the permission of other wives. There is no personal space, or else you will be suspected of something secret. If anything happens to the man, all the wives will be suspected, even if it is the man's fault. If he dies, wives are in trouble because all of us will be suspected as witches. If anything happens to the children too, the wives are in trouble. The mental torture was too much. It was a terrible life.

**Who suspects the wives?**

His family members.

**What do they do after suspecting?**

They can send the wife out and take the children.

**If they are that powerful, why don't they correct the man when he beats his wives?**

The men are always right.

**Probe: So you have to take permission from other wives?**

Yes, if I want to get close to him to share information or ask for something and it is not my day.

**How did you feel about that?**

I felt very unhappy. What kind of life was that?

**Were you trained to expect that in your marriage?**

Yes, but it is still not okay.

**Probe: Tell me more about the plan.**

It is a roster for when to sleep with our husband. Each wife is allotted a day of the week to sleep with him except when the wife is pregnant or nursing. That is one of the reasons why men have more than one wife. When one is pregnant or nursing, another one will be available for sex.

**Did you like the plan?**

I didn't like it at the beginning of my marriage because I wanted to be closer to my husband and I had three days. As years went by, I got used to it, and I was afraid of HIV anyway. So the more the wives, the less the days for each wife, so it was okay with me.

**How did you cope living in polygamy?**

I was afraid that I would catch HIV/AIDS and die because my first husband died of it. I was always praying and watching, and I was rubbing a cream all over my body before sex.

**Probe: Tell me more about the cream.**

It was a cream with menthol. Just to kill any virus or bacteria if they get in contact with my body.

**How did you get the cream?**

I bought it from a witch doctor who was selling it.

**Did you buy it with your own money?**

Yes, I had my own money from the things that I was selling in my shop.

**Did your husband know about it?**

No. We keep such things secret. If he knows, he will accuse me of extramarital affairs and send me away or abandon me in the house.

**Probe: Tell me more about witch doctors.**

They are old people who sell traditional medicine in the community. They are well known and respected.

**Do they do rituals?**

Yes, if they need to do it.

**How do they do rituals?**

I don't know. I only watch them in movies.

**What do you see in movies?**

They take the people to the forest and do incantations. I don't understand the whole thing.

**Did you believe the cream was working?**

Yes, at that time, I believed but not now. I know better now.

**Probe: Do you know better now because you work in health care?**

Yes.

**What was the role of your husband in polygamy?**

He was the master planner. He was the head of the house. He was the decision maker. Nobody can do anything against his wish. He provides for the family.

**You were a trader, which means you were earning money. Did you at any time provide for your family?**

Yes, sometimes for my children, but it is my husband's duty to provide, and he was doing it well.

**Did you provide for other children as well?**

Yes, sometimes.

**Please tell me what you knew then about HIV/AIDS.**

It is a killer disease. It is a death sentence, and people treat you like garbage.

**How do people treat them like garbage?**

By not having anything to do with them. They turn to their family members for a living and go to traditional healers because the hospitals don't treat them.

**Do the traditional healers cure them?**

No.

**Tell me more about what you knew about HIV/AIDS.**

We heard on TV and radio that it comes through sex. Many people died of it then. I and other wives would fight our husband's mistresses and all the prostitutes around because we knew they are the ones who transfer disease around by sleeping with just anybody. We were doing that without our husband's knowledge because, if he knew, he will fight us.

**What were the TV and radio doing?**

They were doing adverts, drama, song, and jingles about HIV/AIDS.

**Were the hospitals also doing anything to alert or educate people?**

Yes, they were distributing flyers.

**Probe: How were you fighting your husband's mistresses and prostitutes?**

We go to warn them to leave our husband alone.

**Probe: How did you identify them?**

We usually watch our husband secretly whenever he was going out, and if we see him often with any lady, we will know something is going on. We will go and warn her, and if she doesn't stop, we will fight her. Young boys in the area also help us to fight them. By that, the prostitutes were running away from our area, and the mistresses were getting married.

**What if your husband goes to them where they ran to?**

I don't think he would go that far for a prostitute.

**What is your opinion about polygamy and HIV/AIDS?**

Polygamy is the vehicle for HIV/AIDS. People go on infecting people and dying everywhere. If they can just listen to the health people and keep to one wife, there will be no HIV.

**Did you see your husband as someone who can keep to one wife?**

No, he was not brought up to know how to keep to one wife.

**How did you perceive your risk for HIV/AIDS when you were in polygamy?**

I knew I was at risk because nobody is faithful to anybody in polygamy and women are a nobody. So we cannot talk. The man outside the marriage with whom the woman satisfies her sexual urges surely must be promiscuous himself. He is therefore a carrier of STDs. But the truth is we women know before we marry that there will be another wife so we know the risk. Some women look forward to having another wife, especially when they start to bear children, knowing that their husband will definitely need to satisfy himself because of their polygamous nature.

**Probe: So you believe that men are polygamous by nature.**

In Africa, men are polygamous by nature.

**Probe: You said nobody is faithful in polygamy. Who is more unfaithful?**

The men are more unfaithful. Women are supposed to be faithful, but when the man cannot satisfy them sexually, they go outside secretly to young boys in the community.

**How did your knowledge of HIV/AIDS affect your sexual relationship with your husband when you were in polygamy?**

We don't use protection, so it was very scary, but as a woman, I have to obey him, and I can't ask for condom if I don't want him to send me out or abandon me. Men are polygamous by nature. He will satisfy himself elsewhere if I don't allow him when it is my turn. I was afraid I would catch HIV. I was not using protection, but I had a cream that I was using to rub my body before intercourse. I got the cream from a witch doctor without my husband's knowledge. If he knew, he would kill me, but I am sure other wives were doing it too. I think it helped because I married him for twelve years and did not have HIV.

**Probe: Was that the same cream with menthol?**

Yes.

**Probe: You said he will abandon you. If he abandons you, where will you go?**

I will go back to my parents, but they will be unhappy because people will blame them for not bringing me up properly.

**Can you remarry?**

I can remarry, but nobody wants to marry a divorced wife.

**Who keeps the children if he sends you out?**

It depends on how old they are and their sex. If they are too young, I keep them. If they are not too young, he keeps them until they are old enough to decide. If they are males, he keeps them. If not, he sends them away with me. He is the owner of the children. He can decide to keep them at any time. That is why we women don't like to divorce.

**Can you take him to court for custody?**

Nobody does that in the village.

**Did you bring all of your children here with you?**

Yes. I won the visa lottery and brought them all.

**How did your husband feel?**

He was happy we were coming here because he thought I will send for him. He was proud his children were going to America.

**Was he proud of you too?**

No, he said he wished he was the one who won the visa lottery. He warned me not to leave him and said, if I leave him, he would curse me. I don't know if he cursed me, but I don't see the curse working because now he is begging me to come here.

**Do the children miss him?**

No, they don't miss him at all.

**How do you know?**

They tell me they don't miss him, but they miss their siblings.

**How is your relationship with your husband in your present marriage where you do not practice polygamy?**

It is heaven on earth. I thank God for bringing me here and meeting my present husband. My past marriage was a mess. My present husband is Nigerian too. He was born here and grew up here. He is a nurse. We spend our money together and love each other.

# INTERVIEW NOTE

**Name**

P4

**What is your age?**

Thirty-nine

**How long have you been in America?**

Six years

**What is your marital status?**

Married

**How long have you been married in America?**

Five years

**What is your present level of education?**

College

**What is your present occupation?**

LPN (licensed practical nurse)

**How old were you when you got married to your husband in Nigeria?**

Twenty-one

**How old was your husband in Nigeria when you got married to him?**

Twenty-three

**Was this your first marriage? And how long?**

Yes. Twelve years.

**What was your education status?**

High school

**What was the education status of your husband?**

High school

**What was your occupation?**

Housewife

**What was the occupation of your husband?**

Teacher

**How many other wives did your husband have, and what were their ages?**

Three other wives. They were younger than me. I don't know their exact ages.

**What was your position among the wives?**

I was the first wife.

**Were other wives taking instructions from you?**

If it had to do with house chores, yes, but our husband is the decision maker for all of us.

**Probe: So you were the most powerful of all the wives.**

Yes, I was, but if our husband shows favoritism, the favorite will be the most powerful at that time, and that is usually the last wife.

**Why was your husband the decision maker?**

That is the culture.

**How many children lived in the home?**

I had four children for him. We don't count other people's children.

**Where are your children now?**

They are all in Nigeria with their father.

**How would you describe your relationship with your husband in Nigeria?**

It was not good at all. It was good at first until he started marrying other women.

**How would you describe the other wives of your husband in Nigeria?**

The second one was not respecting me at first. Later when the third one arrived, she started being nice to me so that I can join her to fight the third one. The third one was very rude. The last one was a bit good. She is very beautiful and always shows off her beauty.

**Tell me about your relationship with other wives.**

We had our good and bad moments. You know there is bound to be quarrels because of the competition and jealousies.

**How often were the quarrels?**

They were always happening.

**Did it involve the children?**

Yes, children sided with their mothers.

**When you quarrel, what was your husband doing about it?**

He did not know about it. We kept it within ourselves just to respect him.

**Probe: If he knew, what would he do?**

He can do anything from scolding to beating.

**When he scolds or beats you, who do you report him to?**

We don't report our husbands. What happens in the home stays in the home. If any wife reports her husband, she will be called a bad wife.

**Probe: If you are injured when he beats you, do you go to hospital?**

No. We treat ourselves at home. If I go to hospital, he will not pay for it, and I am just a housewife who depends on my husband for money.

**Can you divorce him and remarry?**

No, we don't do that in the village because nobody will marry the woman.

**How would you describe your experience of polygamy?**

Polygamy is terrible. What can we do? It is the culture that we were born into, and we women have been taught to accept that our husband will marry more than one wife. No woman likes it, but we have to accept it because we don't have a voice. My experience was not good at all. There was no connection between me and our husband because there were other wives. Our husband had to treat us equally, but it is obvious he loved the last wife.

**How was it obvious?**

He would take her out and be nice to her. Although he was being nice to us all, we knew where his heart was.

**Probe: Were you all jealous of her?**

Yes, but we didn't show it. Or we showed it when our husband was not around.

**How did she react to your jealousy?**

Sometimes she made fun of us. Sometimes she fights.

**Probe: When she fights, is it physical?**

No, it is verbal.

**How did you cope living in polygamy?**

I just minded my own business and kept my attention on my children. I was very unhappy that other wives were competing with me. As for HIV, I was just praying.

**What was the role of your husband in polygamy?**

He was the head of the house. He provided the money that we all spent.

**Were all of the wives housewives?**

Yes, that's what our husband wanted.

**Probe: Why?**

I think it is just to control us. Men do that to control their wives.

**Please tell me what you knew then about HIV/AIDS.**

We were told that HIV was a killer disease.

**Probe: Who told you?**

From the TV and radio. People were dying everywhere in the village. They said the prostitutes were infecting the men and men were bringing it to their wives. I was really afraid, and we started to fight any prostitute we see with our husbands. Who wants to die? The worst part is people were not being sincere about their HIV status for fear of discrimination. Who doesn't want to live a normal life like having a job, wives, and children?

**How were people discriminating against them?**

They were not giving them jobs, housing, anything. Nobody wanted to live them, so they go to their family for help who, in turn, take them to witch doctors for cure.

**Are witch doctors same as traditional healers?**

Yes.

**Do their medicines work for HIV?**

No, the people were dying.

**Probe: Tell me more about prostitutes. When you fight them, how do you do it?**

We would just go to them and warn them to leave our husbands alone, and if they turn it to a fight, we fight them.

**Probe: Is the fight physical or verbal?**

Both. It depends on how they respond.

**Probe: Do all the wives go together to fight the prostitutes?**

Most times, we go together and even bring young area thugs with us to scare them.

**Probe: So you feel that scares them away.**

Yes, it worked. Many of them left our village for the city.

**Can your husband go to them in the city?**

I don't think so, and it never happened with my husband, but if it happens, we would go to the city and fight them.

**So you personally participated in these fights?**

Yes, all of the time.

**What was your husband's reaction?**

He never knew about it. We were doing it secretly. Even if the prostitute tells him, he wouldn't want to confront us with it. It is when wives are caught fighting prostitutes that the husband gets angry and punishes his wives.

**What would he do?**

He can slap or beat us up.

**When he beats you up, do you complain to anybody?**

No, we can't do that. That is like washing your dirty linen in public. Nobody will listen without making fun of you. To the people, he is a real man that disciplines his wives. If you talk about your husband in a negative way, you are a bad wife. There is a popular saying that what happens in the home stays in the home.

**What is your opinion about polygamy and HIV/AIDS?**

I think polygamy is the cause of HIV/AIDS. Men contact it from prostitutes and later give it to their wives. That was why it was spreading like fire. If each man keeps to one wife, it will not spread so much.

**Is it possible for a man to keep to one wife?**

Yes. Africans are the only ones who believe that men are polygamous by nature. What about people in other countries who marry one wife all their lives?

**How did you perceive your risk for HIV/AIDS when you were in polygamy?**

I knew I was at risk for HIV/AIDS and other STDs, but I was just praying. What can I do? Women are not allowed to talk. If we talk, we will be sent packing or abandoned. Who wants to be a single woman that everybody will be cursing? I have witnessed a man marry two wives at a time without any of the wives complaining. The marriage was well celebrated. We can't ask for condom from him. He will get angry and do anything. You know, women are used to these things. Men will always go after girls because of their nature, and we women know that. So we know we are at risk. We just accept whatever comes. The poor economy in Nigeria is forcing men to abandon polygamy little by little. Can you believe that some family members help their men to get wives if they can't afford it? So how would a woman not be at risk?

**Probe: So you knew you were at risk for HIV/AIDS and did not complain.**

Yes, if I complain, he will send me out or abandon me.

**Probe: If he sends you out, where will you go?**

I will have to go back to my poor parents.

**What happens to your children?**

He can decide to keep them if they are boys. If girls, he will send them out with me, and we will become the burden of my family. That is the reason we don't leave.

**How did your knowledge of HIV/AIDS affect your sexual relationship with your husband when you were in polygamy?**

We were just having sex without protection, especially when I was having my children. I can't deny him. That will be against our culture. He has to have it anytime he asks for it. I can't ask for condom if I don't want trouble. At first, sex was for bearing children. Later it turned to once in a while because he wanted it with the younger wives. So the routine did not involve me much. I was happy at that because I was afraid of catching disease. If I catch a disease through him, he will accuse me of bringing the disease. It was just emotionally disturbing to live like that.

**Probe: Tell me more about the routine.**

That is what we call the sex plan. Sex plan is a roster that we do to show who sleeps with him at what day of the week. It is something that we have to keep to; else it turns to a huge fight.

Except the husband changes it. No wife can take another wife's position. It is rare for husbands to change it unless the wife requests for change due to illness or pregnancy. Pregnant and nursing wives don't participate at all.

**How is your relationship with your husband in your present marriage where you do not practice polygamy?**

I really thank God for my present husband. He is Nigerian too, but he is a godly man. He treats me like his best friend. I am truly happy.

**Did you marry for love, family obligation, or another reason?**

I married for love and because I was ready to marry.

**How did you feel about getting married?**

At first, I was happy until the wives started coming one after the other.

**Did your family approve of your prospective husband?**

Yes, they approved of him.

**Did your mother discuss marriages with multiple wives with you?**

Yes, she lectured me about obeying my husband and keeping everything that happens in the home to myself. She said there will always be another wife like we have in my home. My mother is the second wife. She said I should respect my senior wives and be nice to other wives.

**Did your father discuss marriages with multiple wives with you?**

Yes, he always talked about the roles of women and men in the home. He would say the man is the authority man and the decision maker. A woman does not have a voice and should be quiet when the husband is around. She belongs to the man and should not have anything of her own.

**Did you grow up in a city or rural village?**

Rural village.

**If you had grown up in a city, do you believe the issue of marriages with multiple wives would be accepted?**

Yes, it is accepted in the city, but more common in the village.

**Why?**

The city is more civilized, and the people are more educated so they know that with many wives come many STDs.

**Did the multiple wives live in the same house?**

Yes, and every wife has her own room with her children. The husband has a separate room.

**What kind of struggles were there in day-to-day living arrangements with multiple wives and children?**

The children like it because they have many siblings to play with. The wives don't like it because they always fight over everything, like other wives, children, money, space, etc.

**How did you manage the struggles?**

We just lived with it. As a woman, we cannot talk.

**Describe cultural traditions about marriage in some detail. What is the youngest a woman gets married?**

In my village, it is eighteen after high school or thirteen after primary school. It is either through a man meeting a girl and asking her to marry him, and the parents will be notified. Or parents will get together and arrange for their children to meet. In both ways, the man has to pay a bride price before the girl can marry him. The man doesn't need to inform his other wives and children before marrying a new wife, and everybody knows that. The wife is married to the man forever, no divorce except if the woman has extramarital affairs. He will send her back to her parents and curse her. No man will marry her again. This is very rare. Men are the ones who can have extramarital affairs. Women are not allowed to.

**When the man sends the woman out, does he ask for the dowry back?**

If he likes, he can get it back or leave it.

**Can women remain unmarried into their twenties or thirties if she wishes to get advanced education and a career?**

Yes, in the city. No, in the village. I was twenty-one when I got married, and I was considered old.

**Would you ever count the children from other wives as part of your extended family on any level?**

No, we don't.

**Why?**

It is our belief that you might say they are too many, and if anything happens to them, you will be held responsible. That's what I hear the old people say. I don't know how far it is true.

**If one of those other children called you now for help, do you believe you would help him or her?**

Yes, I will.

**How did your children feel about being part of that extended family with other wives and children when you were in Nigeria?**

They liked their siblings, but they don't like that there were many wives.

**Do your adult children ever talk about that part of their lives now? How do they describe their feelings?**

They don't like it because I'm not there with them. They are in Nigeria with their father.

**Why didn't you come here with them?**

He didn't allow them to come with me.

**Are they all males or females?**

They are all males.

**How old are they?**

Seventeen, seventeen, fifteen, and thirteen

**Did you have twins?**

Yes.

**How do you feel not being there with them?**

I don't feel good about it. They are doing well though. I am making arrangements to bring them here.

**Do you feel any influence of Nigerian cultural traditions on your relationships with men in the U.S.?**

No, it is different here. My present husband is Nigerian, but he came here at the age of five so he doesn't know any Nigerian culture.

**Could a wife in a traditional marriage in Nigeria with multiple wives ever refuse sex with her husband?**

No, it can never happen. Women have no choice or voice in anything. They have to allow their husband to do anything with them; else they will be divorced or abandoned.

**What did wives of one husband typically fight about?**

Space is the first thing. No matter how wide the house is, we women always have things like clothes, shoes, or furniture too much for our own space. So when we get into another wife's space, it becomes a fight. Another one is competition for the husband's attention where we cook special meals for the husband after the general meal or dressing up and showing off to attract the husband when he is supposed to be with another wife. The husband can also cause the fight by showing favoritism to one wife by taking her out often, speaking too much about her with friends, or choosing to sleep with her when it is not her turn. Another one is when the husband gives more money to a wife or child of a wife more than others. Money is supposed to be distributed equally unless there is a greater need with a wife or child.

**When you were slapped or caned by your husband, was there anyone you could ever go to for support? For example, a friend or mother?**

No, what happens in the home stays in the home.

**Were there any laws that support a wife who was hurt by her husband? For example, could she ever call the police for support if severely beaten?**

No, we don't call the police. They will support the man, and there is no law supporting the woman.

**In any of the large cities, were there any women's groups that support wives?**

Yes, in the large cities.

**Do you know if there is any current movement to change the cultural tradition of multiple wives?**

Yes, in the city. Some women groups are going against it.

**Please talk a little more about the use of traditional healers in villages versus Western medicine doctors. Do women typically use a traditional healer or Western medicine doctors for pregnancy and childbirth?**

Yes, some women use them while others go to hospital.

**Why?**

Because they are cheaper and the people are more familiar with the traditional healers. They are renowned people who deal in herbs in the village. Their herbs work for most ailments.

**Do the herbs work for HIV/AIDS?**

I don't think so because I have never seen anyone cured of HIV/AIDS by them. People go to them when they are rejected in the hospitals, but the people die eventually.

**What do you think are the benefits of going to a traditional healer versus Western medicine?**

They are cheaper, and the people have more trust and respect for them than Western medicine.

**Do you use them?**

Yes. I use them for headache, fever, body ache, etc. But if I have a chronic illness like diabetes or cancer, I will go to hospital.

**Please discuss your faith traditions in Nigeria. For example, what do priests and pastors say about men having multiple wives?**

In the village, the priests and pastors don't talk about them because they have multiple wives too, but in the city, those of them who don't have multiple wives preach against it. The ones who have keep quiet about it.

**Could a wife in Nigeria go to a priest or pastor for emotional support in dealing with a husband who has multiple wives and girlfriends?**

If the priest or pastor doesn't have multiple wives, yes, and she will be advised to obey her husband and keep calm.

**Could a woman in Nigeria choose college and career over marriage and be accepted?**

Not in the village. Nobody will accept her.

**What will the people do to her?**

Nobody will have anything to do with her. They will treat her with no respect. She will be shamed out of the village. Such things happen only in the city.

**Are girls in Nigeria encouraged to go onto vocational training or university?**

Yes, in the city. But in the village, marriage is the major advice for the woman.

# INTERVIEW NOTE

**Name**

P5

**What is your age?**

Forty-one

**How long have you been in America?**

Seven years

**What is your marital status?**

Married

**How long have you been married in America?**

Six years

**What is your present level of education?**

College

**How many years of college, and what did you study?**

One year. Licensed practical nurse (LPN)

**Did you graduate?**

Yes.

**What is your present occupation?**

LPN (Licensed practical nurse)

**How old were you when you got married in Nigeria?**

I was twenty-one.

**How old was your husband when you got married to him in Nigeria?**

He was twenty-one too.

**Was this your first marriage? And how long?**

Yes. Thirteen years.

**Was the marriage arranged?**

No.

**How did you meet?**

We met in high school. He used to sit by me and teach me in school. When we were in Class 3 of high school, he told me he wanted me to be his girlfriend. I accepted because I liked him too. Our friends and classmate knew about us, but we kept it from our parents.

**What would your parents do?**

They would stop us because we were still in school. Parents are afraid that their female children will be pregnant if she had a boyfriend while in school.

**What would they do if you were pregnant?**

I will not be allowed in school anymore, and that will be a shame on my parents because, when such thing happens, people will blame parents for not bringing their daughter up properly.

**What about the boy?**

He has no blame. He will continue with his studies.

**So that is why you kept your relationship from your parents?**

Yes.

**What was your education status in Nigeria?**

High school

**What was the education status of your husband in Nigeria?**

High school

**What was your occupation in Nigeria?**

Ward maid (LNA)

**What was the occupation of your husband in Nigeria?**

Hospital clerk

**How many other wives did your husband have, and what were their ages?**

Two other wives, but one died. I don't know their ages.

**Why did your husband marry another wife?**

Men marry more than one wife in Nigeria to boost their ego. They are proud that they have many wives that they are controlling. It also shows that they have money.

**How do they marry the wives?**

They either approach the girl and talk to her or go to her parents, who will then ask the girl to marry him. Sometimes the present wife looks for another wife for the husband, like in my own case. I brought the second wife for my husband. He chose the third one by himself. When the second one died, I brought a fourth one, but he refused.

**Why did he refuse?**

He said he didn't want any more.

**Can a girl refuse to marry a man chosen for her by her parents or anybody?**

Yes, if her parents allow her to refuse. If not, she has to marry him because, before they consult her, they must have taken money from the man.

**Can they return the money if she refuses?**

No, they don't return such money. It is the dowry so the girl has to marry him.

**What if she runs away?**

They will catch her and bring her back.

**What was your position among the wives?**

The first wife

**How did you feel as each wife came?**

I was okay with it. We women already know that will happen, so we are prepared.

**Did you know the wives before they came?**

No. None of them was from our community.

**Were you the one giving instructions to the wives?**

Yes, when it has to do with keeping the house. Other instructions came from our husband. The last wife sometimes assumes authority if our husband allows her to claim the favorite wife.

**Why would your husband give instruction or allow the favorite wife?**

That is the culture.

**Probe: Tell me more about the culture**

The first wife gives instruction on shopping for foodstuff and other items for the home. Usually the last wife is the favorite until a new wife comes in. At the time, she is the favorite. Our husband can give her information to pass to us, such as when he will come back from work or the type of food he wants to eat for dinner. Our husband is the decision maker when it comes to providing money for the home and the children's school.

**Probe: So you believe this order should be followed in marriage?**

That was how it was handed down to us. I saw my father and his numerous wives do it.

**How many children lived in the home?**

I had four, and my co-wives had children too that I cannot count according to culture.

**So the culture forbids counting other people's children.**

Yes, we believe that comes from the Bible where David counted the Israelites and they died.

**Where are your children now?**

Two older ones are in Nigeria. My first child is married in Nigeria and living her life. My second lives with her. Two younger ones are here with me.

**How old are they?**

Nineteen, eighteen, fifteen, and fifteen

**Probe: You had a set of twins?**

Yes, both are boys.

**How did you bring them here?**

Through relatives here.

**Did you leave them with your husband when you were coming here?**

Yes.

**Did he resist when relatives were bringing two of them here?**

No, it's a thing of pride to our men that they have children abroad. The wives are the ones that they don't allow to travel abroad because they know the woman's eyes will open and she will not come back to them.

**When she doesn't come back to them, how do they feel?**

They feel bad. Some of them resort to telling people that the wife has become a prostitute in America, while others will be begging the wife to come and take them to America.

**If your husband begs you to come and bring him here, will you accept?**

No. I will not. I am married to somebody else. I don't want a polygamist in my life anymore.

**Were your children happy coming here, and do they miss their father?**

They were very happy coming here. None of them has ever told me they miss their father. They were always telling me they missed me when they were in Nigeria.

**Do you know why they didn't miss him?**

They enjoy this place more. They only miss the food and nature in Nigeria.

**How would you describe your relationship with your husband in Nigeria?**

Not really much. He was my husband and the father of my children. Nothing much. It's not like here where husband and wife love each other and take decisions together. No, the husband's word is law in Nigeria. We didn't have much connection because there were other wives.

**Is there a rule regarding husband and wife not loving each other?**

No. Men do it to show that they are strong men who don't show emotions, and they also do it so that wives don't feel jealous.

Some men can decide to show love to one wife to make others jealous, and the wives will be fighting one another.

**How did your children feel when they knew you were not loved by their father or when another wife comes in?**

They didn't know at that time that we didn't love each other. Children don't know their fathers don't love their mothers. The male child is tutored by his father not to show love to his wives so as to appear as a strong man. The girls are tutored to obey their husbands and know there will be other wives. The children accept another wife into the family each time they came. They don't have to know before the wives come. Our husband never prepared any of his children for that. They have no choice.

**Was he preparing you wives by telling you ahead that another wife was coming?**

No, he would just bring her and announce to the whole family.

**How did you feel about that?**

I didn't feel anything at that time, but when I think back now, I feel angry.

**How would you describe the other wives of your husband in Nigeria?**

The second one was good, but she had her bad sides, like gossiping and competing with me to court our husband's favor by cooking and dressing up for our husband. It's a pity she died in an accident. The other wife was the third wife. She was always fighting, and she liked to show off everything she had.

She was a ward maid (LNA) like me. She was a liar of the first order. She would always cook up stories that my husband fell for, and there was always chaos in the house. She loves it when everybody is fighting everybody.

**Who was she fighting?**

Me and the other wife.

**How was she fighting?**

She would shout and call us all sorts of names, and when people talked to her to stop, she will call them names too.

**When your husband fell for her lies, what would he do?**

He would scold us for her.

**How did you feel about that?**

I felt very unhappy each time it happened, but I would just keep quiet.

**Tell me about your relationship with other wives.**

It was not good at all. We were always fighting.

**Were you fighting one another or your husband and children?**

No, we were not fighting our husband and children. We fought each other.

**Probe: When you fought, was it physical or verbal?**

It was verbal.

**How did your husband react to the fight?**

He would just order us to keep quiet, but when it gets too much, he would leave the house for us. Most times we fought in his absence and kept a straight face in his presence so that he will not leave the house.

**Probe: How do the children react to the fights?**

They usually side with their mothers.

**When children side with their mothers, do you wives talk to the other wife's children to make them see reason?**

Sometimes we do that, and the children tries to settle the wives.

**How were the children getting along?**

They play, eat, and do things together.

**How would you describe your experience of polygamy?**

Not good at all. If I come back to life, I will not go to any place where they practice polygamy. There is no freedom, no enjoyment. The man was just not there. He was busy chasing his mistresses all about. Though I know men are polygamous by nature, they should at least love their wives, but no, there is no love in polygamy. Only planned sex where you take turns. You dare not take another wife's place. The husband will enjoy it because that is double enjoyment for him, but the wives will fight to finish.

**What do you mean by men are polygamous by nature?**

That is our belief in Africa, but I have seen that African men are the only ones polygamous by nature in Africa. Outside Africa, they are not polygamous. I am married to an African man here, and he has never been polygamous.

**Can you stop him from chasing his mistresses all about?**

No, we can't do that.

**Why?**

He will be offended and do it more.

**To spite you?**

Yes, and to make me jealous.

**Probe: Can't you stop the mistresses?**

We do when we know them.

**How were you stopping them?**

We would go to them with area boys and warn them to stop seeing our husband.

**Does it get physical?**

It gets physical sometimes so as to shame the mistresses. These mistresses are prostitutes, and because they are not respected in the society, people join wives to fight them when such fights occur.

**How did your husband react to the fight?**

We were doing it without his knowledge.

**Probe: Tell me more about planned sex.**

It is a roster that we make to show the days when each wife would sleep with the husband. When we were three, we used to make it a daily affair. My days were Mondays and Tuesdays, the second wife Wednesdays and Thursdays, and the third wife Fridays, Saturdays, and Sundays. The last wife usually has more days because she is the most recent wife and needs to enjoy the husband more. When the second wife died and our husband refused to marry another one to replace her, I took her Wednesdays, and the third wife took her Thursdays. When one of us is pregnant, nursing, or menstruating, it is enjoyment galore for the other wives because the wife is excluded from the roster.

**How did you cope living in polygamy?**

I was just praying. It is good that we were not many, but if there is disease, my husband would put it on one of us. Men don't admit that they have disease. I was afraid, but I can't talk as a woman. Our culture doesn't give women a voice. I had to let him do whatever he wanted to do.

**When the men get seriously sick, do they admit that they have disease?**

Yes, and they blame their wives for the disease.

**Probe: Even when it is a chronic disease like diabetes?**

Yes, they say it is the wife who gave them wrong food to eat. When it is infectious, they say it is the wife who infected them.

**Has that ever happened to you?**

Yes, he was sick with typhoid fever and told everybody we gave him dirty water to drink, and when we explained to him it was not infected water, he shouted on us and accused us of trying to kill him.

**How was he treated?**

He went to the traditional healer in the village.

**Was he cured?**

Yes.

**Probe: So you believe in traditional medicine.**

Yes, the medicine man is a herbalist. They deal in African herbs that cure diseases.

**Do you believe they can cure HIV/AIDS?**

I think they are still looking for a herb that cures HIV because I have not seen anyone cured by them.

**Do they perform rituals, and do you think, if they perform rituals, they might find a cure?**

Yes, they perform rituals. I am sure they must have performed rituals without finding a cure.

**When they perform rituals, what do they do?**

They and their clients are the ones who know about that.

**Have you ever had that experience?**

No.

**What was the role of your husband in polygamy?**

He was the head of the house. He was our decision maker. He provided money for the home.

**Probe: You were a working wife as well as one other wife. Can both of you spend your money to provide for the family?**

No, the man provides for the family. In my home, all our money goes into one account. Our husband was in charge of everything. He dictates how money is spent.

**Probe: Even your own money?**

Yes, if I complain, he can stop me from working. It is a privilege that he allowed us to work so he has to be in control of the money. We were not allowed to spend money without his consent.

**Please tell me what you knew then about HIV/AIDS.**

They said it was a killer disease without cure.

**Probe: Who said that?**

The TV and radio people. The hospital staff too.

**Were they making advertisements?**

Yes, they were doing stories, drama, and songs, and the hospital workers were going from house to house to distribute flyers and speak with the people. It was a death sentence if you have it. So many people died from it. Once you get it and declare it, you are tagged. Nobody comes near you. Those who had it were going to traditional healers because the hospitals were rejecting them. The men were catching it from having sex with many girls. I was always telling my children not to have sex because of HIV. One of my brothers died of it.

**Did you use traditional healers for him?**

Yes.

**Did the medicine work?**

No. I was going into my brother's house to care for him when he was down with AIDS until he died. His numerous wives and children abandoned him because they did not want to catch the disease.

**Why didn't you take him to the hospital?**

Hospital workers don't accept them. They said they cannot cure them, and they were afraid of catching the disease too.

**What is your opinion about polygamy and HIV/AIDS?**

Polygamy is the reason there is so much HIV in Nigeria. Men were infecting their wives because there is no faithfulness in polygamy. Women are taught to be ready for polygamy because men are polygamous by nature. It is a thing of pleasure to them; it boosts their ego. African men love to boast of their numerous wives.

**Probe: You said there is no faithfulness in polygamy. Does this apply to both men and women?**

The women are supposed to be faithful not the men. Most women are faithful until there are too many wives and mistresses and the husband is not available anymore or they are not able to satisfy all the wives sexually.

**Probe: What would the women do at that point?**

They go secretly to young boys in the community for sexual satisfaction. They buy gifts for the boys so that they can keep it secret. If they don't have money to buy gifts, they take food from the house to them. Some women are afraid to do it because of the curse of death attached to it, but others don't really care about the curse.

**Probe: Do you believe in the curse?**

I used to believe it, but not anymore.

**Probe: Why don't you believe it anymore?**

Because it doesn't make sense to me anymore.

**How did you perceive your risk for HIV/AIDS when you were in polygamy?**

I knew I was at risk from the moment I saw my husband going about with girls, but I received a thorough lesson on how to be in good relationship with my husband. Any woman who thinks her husband is not seeing another woman is deceiving herself. In fact, some women even prefer to choose the wife for their husbands so that the husband will not go and bring a woman who will be fighting them. I know I was at risk of contracting HIV, but I was lucky that my husband allowed me to choose wives for him. Apart from the fact that they were fighting and competing, they were faithful to our husband to the best of my knowledge.

**If they were not faithful, can you tell on them?**

No, they will arrange my downfall. I can only talk to them to be careful. Thank God I didn't have that experience.

**How did your knowledge of HIV/AIDS affect your sexual relationship with your husband when you were in polygamy?**

In my thirteen years of marriage to him, he never used condom. He always said he hated it like hell. That means to me that he has tried it outside the marriage. Inside the marriage, no wife dares mention it. Apart from that, I had to have children, especially a male child, if I want to stay married to him. My first two were females, and I know they don't have any inheritance in the home. If my husband dies, I will be sent out with my daughters so I was just allowing my husband to impregnate me. Protection did not come up at all even after I stopped having children. That is something a woman cannot ask for if you don't want to leave or be abandoned. You just have to obey him. I was living in fear. I hated it so much, but I have to let him when it is my turn.

**Probe: Fear of what?**

Fear of HIV, abandonment, beating, or even death.

**If you fear so much, why did you not leave him?**

No, I couldn't leave him. Our culture forbids women leaving their husbands. No man will marry a divorced woman, and my children will suffer without me.

**If he sends you out, where will you go?**

I will go back to my parents' house.

**Probe: With your children?**

No, he will not allow the children to follow me. They are his children, not mine, except the female ones.

**What if the children refuse to stay with him?**

Unless they are old enough not to depend on him, they cannot decide that. Else he will disown them. He can let go of the girls, but the boys definitely stay with him. It is because of all the troubles that we women stay in the marriage despite all the risks of diseases or even death.

**Can you take him to court and sue for custody if he takes your children?**

There is no court for that in the village. The man is the owner of the children.

**Probe: You mentioned beating. When your husband beats you, do you go to hospital for treatment?**

No. We treat ourselves at home because we can't pay hospital bills, and he will definitely not pay.

**Do people come to your rescue when he beats you?**

Yes, they pacify him, but they put all the blame on the wife.

**Can you report him to somebody in his family or community members?**

We don't bother to involve people because they will call us names like "bitches, bad wives talking ill of their husbands, etc." What happens in our home stays in our home.

**How is your relationship with your husband in your present marriage where you do not practice polygamy?**

Perfect. There is love and freedom of speech. We both attend church, and we are happy together. He works as an accountant, and we spend our money together. I have no child with him because he doesn't want children. He accepts my children as his children. It is his second marriage. The first was in Nigeria with no child, and the wife left him for another man with whom she had a son. He relocated here ten years ago.

# INTERVIEW NOTE

**Name**

P6

**What is your age?**

Eighteen

**How long have you been in America?**

One year

**What is your marital status?**

Single but formerly married. In a relationship.

**What is your present level of education?**

High school

**What is your present occupation?**

Unemployed

**How old were you when you got married in Nigeria?**

Sixteen years

**How old was your husband when you got married to him in Nigeria?**

Fifty-five years

**Was this your first marriage? And how long?**

Yes. One year.

**Was it arranged?**

Yes. He was my father's friend.

**How was it arranged?**

He told my father he was interested in me and paid him money.

**Is that money the bride price, the dowry?**

Yes.

**What other things did he give your father, apart from money?**

I don't know of other things. I'm pretty sure money was the major thing. On the day of the marriage, he brought food and drinks for the people and clothes for me.

**Did you like the arrangement?**

No.

**Could you run away?**

No, I didn't want to shame my parents, and I liked my husband.

**Probe: Despite the age difference?**

Yes, he was very nice to me. He used to give me money and buy clothes for me. I was the favorite wife, and he was taking me out all the time I was with him. He did not treat me harshly. I was happy with him.

**Were other wives jealous of you?**

I think so. They always say I am beautiful. If they were jealous, they didn't show it much. They were nice to me, but I was afraid they were pretending.

**Why do you think they were pretending?**

When co-wives talk about the other wife's beauty, that is jealousy.

**Is that the belief?**

Yes. Women say that to their co-wives when they feel they are not as beautiful as the co-wife.

**Probe: And you were afraid of that?**

Yes. If I am not nice to them, out of jealousy, they can tell a lie on me to our husband, and he will send me out.

**Where will you go if that happens?**

Back to my parents.

**What will happen to all the money he paid?**

They will send me back if they can't pay back his money. He will let me live with him, but he will abandon me. He will not touch me for anything.

**Did that happen to you or any of the wives?**

No.

**Did your husband tell the wives and children about you before he brought you in?**

I don't think he had to do that. My father never told us and his wives that he was bringing a new wife.

**Do you think that was why they were jealous?**

No, that was not an expectation. We women know there will be other wives.

**What was your education status in Nigeria?**

I did not finish high school.

**Why?**

I was not really serious with school at that time.

**What was the education status of your husband?**

None. He was illiterate.

**Did you ask him why?**

Yes, he said he had money because his family was rich so he did not need school. Besides his parents didn't go to school as well.

**What was your occupation?**

Housewife

**What was the occupation of your husband?**

Business

**What kind of business?**

Transportation and car dealership

**How many other wives did your husband have, and what were their ages?**

Four other wives. I don't know their ages. Nobody talked about age. They were all older than me.

**What was your position among the wives?**

The last wife

**Were you taking instructions from the senior wives?**

It depends on what we were doing. If it is about taking care of the house and our husband likes cleaning and cooking, yes, I was taking instruction from all of them. Our husband gave the orders for other things.

**Other things such as what?**

Such as the children, their school fees, and how many is spent.

**How was money spent?**

Our husband was giving us money for food and each one of us for personal expenses every week.

**Why was your husband the only one responsible for making money decisions? Can the wives work and earn their own money?**

It is the culture.

**Tell me about what you mean by culture.**

We believe that the husband is the head of the house. He has to provide the money to spend if he wants to keep his authority as the man. Men marry many wives to show off their wealth because, if they don't have money, they cannot marry many wives. My husband does not believe in women working and spending their own money. If we bring money home as gifts or from our parents before marriage, everything belongs to him. We have to give the money to him, and he can give us on a monthly basis as we need it.

**How do you feel about that?**

I used to feel good about it. That was how we were brought up. Men and women are taught their roles in marriage.

**How many children lived in the home?**

Many children

**How did they get along?**

Pretty well. Playing together and sharing things among themselves. They don't quarrel.

**How would you describe your relationship with your husband in Nigeria?**

He liked me being the youngest wife. I was afraid of that because I saw that other wives were not happy. I liked him for taking care of me. I would have preferred him as my husband, not our husband.

**How would you describe the other wives of your husband in Nigeria?**

They were nice but were always competing with one another. Sometimes they fight.

**How did they compete?**

Dressing up for our husband and cooking special dishes for him apart from the general dish. They were doing it so that he will take them out and boast about them.

**Who cooks the general dish?**

I did as the last wife. Older children join me too.

**How did you feel doing that much cooking?**

Oh, I love to cook.

**When wives fight, was it physical?**

No, it was verbal, like calling each other names and shouting on each other.

**Was it a continuous thing or just when a new wife comes?**

It is a continuous thing from when a new wife comes. It never stops.

**What was your husband's reaction to the fights?**

He never knew about it. They did it secretly.

**Tell me about your relationship with other wives.**

They were nice to me, and I was nice to them. Although there was competition here and there and verbal abuses among them, they did not extend it to me because I was like a child to them. Our husband's first three children are older than me. I am same age as his fourth child so my co-wives treated me like their child, and I was nice to them too.

**How would you describe your experience of polygamy?**

I did not really like it, though my husband was nice to me. There was too much competition. Everybody wanted to have the man to themselves. Then there was the fear of catching a disease. Then there was a plan we had to follow to sleep with the man. It was just annoying, but that was the culture, and we women are used to it.

**There was fear of disease? Why when the man was faithful?**

He was getting old. He may not be satisfying the women sexually so they can secretly have a boyfriend.

**How would they do that?**

They will look for young boys around and give them money and gifts so that they can be their boyfriends until they have their own wife. It is all done in secret as long as they keep giving the boy money and gifts.

**How did the wives get money to give boys and to dress up?**

I think they were taking it from money for food. Our husband usually gave money for food every week. He would put it in a particular place for us to spend for the week and then give each one of us and each child money to spend for our personal upkeep for a week. The money for personal upkeep is not much so I don't know how else they get money to buy clothes and jewelries if not from food money, which was really much at that time.

**How did you cope living in polygamy?**

I was just hoping that I will not have the disease, and thank God I didn't. I was praying anytime it was my turn to have sex with my husband. We did not use protection. I wanted a child with him, but I was afraid of HIV. I was using protection with my boyfriend though. I didn't want to bring disease to my husband.

**Probe: So you had a boyfriend?**

Yes. It was a secret. I needed a young man. My marriage was arranged.

**Tell me more about your boyfriend.**

I knew him in high school. If my parents had not arranged my marriage, I would have married him. We could not leave each other even after my marriage because we were in the same community.

**Do you know if he is married now?**

I have not heard about him since I came here.

**Were you afraid your husband would discover?**

Yes, but we both kept it secret.

**What would he do if he discover?**

He would send me out and place a curse on me. Nobody will ever marry me. We believe women with such experience die young mysteriously.

**Will your parents take you back and pay the dowry back?**

No, in that case, they won't even come near me because it is a shame to them, and my husband won't go near them or ask for his money.

**Now that you have left your husband, is he still friends with your father?**

No, they don't fight, but their friendship is not as close as it used to be, and no money is retuned.

**What was the role of your husband in polygamy?**

He was the authority man. He did not use authority much though. He is a nice man, and he was providing very well for us.

**Please tell me what you knew then about HIV/AIDS.**

We heard it is a killer disease. The TV and radio was always talking about it.

**How?**

They were doing adverts and drama. They said you get it through having sex with different people. The prostitute business was not moving anymore in the village because the wives were fighting them. When you get it, the next thing is death because it has no cure. People were dying a lot in the village. The people who had it were keeping it secret so that other people will not reject them. Honestly it was a terrible disease. The best way to prevent it is to keep to one partner who doesn't have it. My brother died of it. We never knew if he were having sex, but we suspected he was. How else could he have got it? Was the question then, but now I know better.

**Probe: How do you know better?**

I am surrounded by nurses who give me proper health education.

**Were people actually rejecting people who had HIV?**

Yes, people were running away from them, including hospital workers. It was their family who was taking care of them and also paying witch doctors to take care of them. Same thing happened with my brother.

**Who are witch doctors?**

They are traditional healers in the town.

**Did they cure the people?**

No.

**So you took your brother there when you suspected he had HIV?**

Yes, when he refused to tell us what was wrong with him, we took him to one.

**Did he cure him?**

No, he died the week he got there.

**How did you know it was HIV and not something else?**

The witch doctor told us he confessed to him that he had been diagnosed of HIV.

**You talked about wives fighting prostitutes. Did you participate in the fights?**

No. My husband did not have mistresses, but I saw women fighting their husbands' mistresses. Some of the mistresses were prostitutes.

**Probe: Tell me what you witnessed.**

The wives would arrange with area boys and go to the prostitutes' house to beat them up or just warn them to leave their husband alone.

**Did their husbands know about it?**

No, they did it secretly.

**Do you know why?**

Yes, some men can side with the prostitute and punish their wives for it.

**What kind of punishment?**

They can beat their wives up in turn.

**Do you know if the wives go to hospital for treatment?**

No, they cannot go to hospital. Where would they get the money to pay? Even if they are working, their money goes into the husband's account.

**Can they report their husband to elders in the community?**

No woman will report her husband. She will be labelled as a bad wife. What happens in the house stays in the house.

**What is your opinion about polygamy and HIV/AIDS?**

Polygamy is just the thing that spreads HIV/AIDS. One person gets HIV and passes it over to another person, who then passes it over to another person. It's just crazy. The women cannot ask the men to use condom. The men will beat the hell out of them because it is like suspecting the man of having a disease.

**Don't men have diseases?**

They don't admit that they have disease. If he is infected, he will put it on his wife, even if he is promiscuous.

**Did you have that experience with your husband?**

No, he was a faithful man.

**Has he ever been sick of any type of disease and put it on you, his wives?**

Yes, when he had malaria, he said we opened the doors for mosquito. When he had typhoid, he said we gave him infected water.

**What happens when the wife is sick?**

He would say the wife brought it on herself.

**How did you perceive your risk for HIV/AIDS when you were in polygamy?**

I know I was at risk, but I was trained to obey my husband. Besides, he was not my only man because he was too old to satisfy me, so I had a boyfriend outside. You see, that is how HIV spreads. When I married a man as old as my father, I expected I would meet some wives there, and I knew I was not going to be the last one. That is the men's nature, and it makes them proud. All of us were at risk of HIV/AIDS, but because we are used to the custom, we don't think about the risk at all. I was in constant fear. There was too much competition among the wives. Sex and other things were used to attract our husband, and I could not complain for fear of being abandoned. When I couldn't bear it anymore, I sought help from a friend who lived in the city, who told me about the female condom. But then my husband was very rich, and I wanted to have a child for him. He was also very nice to me and other wives. He never went out of the marriage to have sex, but I don't trust other wives. When I won the American visa lottery, I fled. Thank God I had no child for him.

**Probe: You don't trust them because they could have a boyfriend like you?**

Yes.

**How did your knowledge of HIV/AIDS affect your sexual relationship with your husband when you were in polygamy?**

Sex was a planned thing. This was the most frustrating for me. Though I was afraid of catching HIV, I was also looking to have a child with him. I trusted him because he was not running after girls. He was just observing the culture. The other wives were the ones that I don't trust. I have a feeling they too were seeing other men. The wives are the ones who bring in the disease.

**Observing the culture how?**

By having many wives. That is what Nigerian men do.

**Is it the wives or the husbands who bring in disease?**

Both of them if they are not faithful.

**Probe: Tell me about the planned sex.**

We had a roster for when to sleep with our husband. Each wife goes to sleep with him on her own day. At the time I came, the first wife was not participating in it because, according to our husband, she was too old for sex. Later I learned that she was abandoned because she asked our husband about condom and he started suspecting her. That left four of us for seven days. I got three days being the youngest and newest wife. The fourth wife had two days, and the rest had a day each. Any of us who was pregnant or menstruating would give up her place to one of the other wives.

**Probe: Was the plan causing fight and competition because the days were not evenly distributed?**

No, it is a routine that we all agreed to.

**Who makes the plan?**

All of us and our husband.

**Probe: Were you all happy with the plan?**

I was not happy with the plan at all, and I'm not sure other wives were happy with it as well. Though I had three days, it was not something that I enjoyed doing. I just wanted to have a child for him, but I didn't have any.

**How is your relationship with your husband in your present marriage where you do not practice polygamy?**

I don't have one yet. My present boyfriend loves me, and I love him too. We are planning to get married soon. He is an African American. He works at the hospital, and he paid for me to do my GED, which I passed very well. He wants to go back to school for health informatics while I do human services. When I become his wife, I can say this is my husband, not our husband.

# INTERVIEW NOTE

**Name**

P7

**What is your age?**

Forty-five

**How long have you been in America?**

Five years

**What is your marital status?**

Widowed

**What is your present level of education?**

High school

**What is your present occupation?**

Clothing business

**How old were you when you got married?**

Nineteen

**How old was your husband when you got married to him?**

Twenty-one

**Was this your first marriage? And how long?**

Yes. Twenty-one years.

**What was your education status?**

High school, but did not finish.

**What was the education status of your husband?**

Primary school

**What was your occupation?**

Housewife

**What was the occupation of your husband?**

Transport business

**How many other wives did your husband have, and what were their ages?**

Five other wives. They were all younger than me.

**What was your position among the wives?**

First wife

**Probe: Were other wives taking instructions from you?**

Yes, for household chores. Other decisions come from our husband.

**Why your husband?**

It is the culture.

**Did he have a favorite among you who can also give instructions?**

Yes, he picks any of us as the favorite at any time.

**How many children lived in the home?**

Many children. I had one girl.

**Where is she now?**

She is here in the U.S.

**How did she come here?**

She won the visa lottery and came here.

**How would you describe your relationship with your husband in Nigeria?**

Nothing good about it. We did not have a relationship apart from being the father of my child.

**How would you describe the other wives of your husband in Nigeria?**

They were wicked and terrible. When they first come, they would be nice. Once they start having children, they show their true colors. Terrible women.

**Tell me about your relationship with other wives.**

We were always fighting. Too much lies and competition.

**Was it physical fight or verbal?**

It was both.

**When you fight physically, do people come around to separate you?**

Yes.

**What did your husband do about it?**

Nothing. He would just leave the house for us because sometimes he caused the fight.

**How did he cause fights?**

By showing favoritism through gifts or anyhow.

**When he caused the fight, can you report him to his family members?**

No, we don't talk about our husband. It is wrong in our culture. We keep everything that happens in our family to ourselves.

**When you are injured in a fight, do you go to hospital?**

No, we treat ourselves at home.

**Probe: Why? Will he not pay the bills?**

No, he will never pay such bills.

**Can you pay the bills?**

No, we don't have our own money. He never allowed us to work so he can control us. He gave us money for everything when he felt like. When he didn't feel like, he would leave us in hunger for days and go after the prostitutes.

**How do you get money for food when he left you to care for yourself and others?**

I turn to friends and family members.

**Why did you stay in the marriage?**

If I leave, the society will blame me, and no man will marry me. It is a bad label in our society to be a single woman. Then my only child will suffer because he will not allow her to leave so as to punish me. Though she is a girl, it doesn't matter with my husband as long as it will make me feel bad.

**Would your family take care of you if you leave?**

Yes, I have a strong family. We take care of one another. It was my brother who helped me and my child to be here today.

**But your child won the visa lottery?**

Yes, my brother paid for the ticket.

**How would you describe your experience of polygamy?**

It was terrible. There was nothing called love in that marriage. There was a plan for sex that nobody can go against, or else there will be trouble. You go in to the man when it is your turn for sex. Just have sex and bear children. Nobody cares about anybody. Too many children fighting and mothers taking sides. Mothers fighting and children taking sides too. Wives are in competition all the time, and they are cheating because the husband cannot satisfy all of them. Usually I as the first wife bears everything. I would just keep quiet and watch all of them do all the mess. If I talk, my husband can join them against me and accuse me of jealousy and other things. But when any of the wives come near me and start a fight, I fight them to finish.

**Did the fight ever stop at any point?**

It never stopped.

**How were the wives cheating?**

They had secret boyfriends in the area that they give gifts.

**But they don't have money. How do they buy gifts for their boyfriends?**

They take from the foodstuff money or cook for them from the household food.

**Did your husband know?**

No, they do it secretly. If he knows, he will send them away after beating them publicly and placing a curse on them.

**How did you cope living in polygamy?**

I was just expecting anything at any time. I was praying and hoping that I would not catch disease. Thank God that my prayer was answered. I would have died with all of them.

**Probe: Did they all die?**

Our husband died of HIV. Some of the wives are sick in hospital now, and the hospital is in the city, far from our village. The hospital in our village doesn't take people with HIV. The village people also don't have anything to do with them. The family is the one who takes care of them, and the care is not that much.

**What was the role of your husband in polygamy?**

He was the head of the house, decision maker, and everybody feared him. He was the one responsible for providing the money that we all spent.

**Please tell me what you knew then about HIV/AIDS.**

It is a killer disease that men get from having sex with girls who have it because those girls who have it don't tell the men so that the men will not run away from them.

**Does that mean people were not having anything to do with them?**

Yes, except their family and their traditional healers because the hospital doesn't take them too.

**Does the medication from traditional healers cure them?**

No, they end up dying within a few months.

**Tell me more about your knowledge of HIV in Nigeria.**

The TV and radio people were telling people to be careful because it was killing people all around both in the village and city. At first, we thought it was a disease of the city people because we were hearing about people dying of it in the city. Later, we started seeing people around us in the village dying of AIDS, and the hospital workers were saying HIV, the "killer disease," is at it again anytime they gave the news of the death to the family. The men were bringing it to their wives, and the wives too are getting it by having boyfriends with their husbands. I was afraid because I have just one daughter. I was always watching out for her. I didn't want the boys to come near her at all.

**What is your opinion about polygamy and HIV/AIDS?**

Polygamy is the father of HIV/AIDS. If there is no polygamy, there will be no HIV. The TV and radio people caution our people to have just one partner, but they did not listen. All these men claim their polygamy nature to flirt around and have many wives. Then they started falling sick and dying. Don't blame them; blame the culture. If the men don't do it, the people will not respect them, but when they cannot satisfy all their wives, the wives will start to have boyfriends and bring disease into the house. The younger wives do this a lot and even go for their husband's older children secretly so that, if they get pregnant, the child will look like their husband. We all knew this was happening. Very shameful.

**How did you perceive your risk for HIV/AIDS when you were in polygamy?**

I was at risk, but what can I do as a woman? It is against the culture to say no to your husband if you don't want trouble. He can send you out or abandon you. We have been brought up to know they will have more than one wife because of their nature. My marriage was a perfect one until the wives started arriving year after year. Before long, I was forgotten. I couldn't complain. You know women cannot say anything but "Thank God that I didn't get HIV." My husband eventually came down with HIV and some of the wives too. Oh! God bless the children. I don't know what has become of them. I had to come over here with my only child that I had for him as soon as I had the opportunity. The wives were always fighting, and our husband would leave the house as a form of punishment for us. Sometimes, he would go for weeks, and we will have to welcome him with open arms if we don't want him to go back. What a shame! Thank God I am not in that mess anymore. He died a few years ago.

**How did your knowledge of HIV/AIDS affect your sexual relationship with your husband when you were in polygamy?**

There was nothing I could do. We were just doing it to obey him, but I was afraid of HIV/AIDS because there was no protection. If I ask for protection, he will start suspecting me, and that is trouble. It is enough ground for divorce. One of my co-wives was sent packing because she told our husband to use condom before sex with her. Our husband said she must have been using it with other men. I was always thinking of what to do so I will not catch the disease when it is my turn on the roster. Sometimes

I would pray; sometimes I will pretend I was sick. Everything was just irritating. In the end, he left me alone because he said I was getting old and he had younger wives. I was happy secretly.

**Probe: Any prescription from anybody like medical doctors or witch doctors?**

No.

**How is your relationship with your husband in your present marriage where you do not practice polygamy?**

No husband. In a relationship with a white American who loves me totally. We do things together. No controlling and selfishness.

**Did you marry for love, family obligation, or another reason?**

I married for both love and family obligation. I loved my husband at first sight when I met him. It was at a time that my parents were also telling me it was time to get married because I had dropped from high school.

**How did you feel about getting married?**

I liked it at first but later discovered my husband was incapable of love.

**Did you talk to him about it?**

When I confronted him with it, he shouted on me.

**Did your family approve of your prospective husband?**

Yes.

**Did your mother discuss marriages with multiple wives with you?**

Yes, she would always tell me about the things I saw in our home while growing up, like how my father married many wives and how the wives must obey him even when he was wrong.

**How did your father marry his wives?**

He was just bringing them home and introducing them to all of us, and that's it. Nobody queries him.

**Did your father discuss marriages with multiple wives with you?**

Yes. He was always talking about the roles of husband and wives in the home, like the wife is the one who cooks, cleans, takes care of the children, and sleeps with the husband when it is her turn. The husband is the decision maker and provider of money for the home.

**Did you grow up in a city or rural village?**

I grew up in the rural village in Beere, Ibadan.

**If you had grown up in a city, do you believe the issue of marriages with multiple wives would be accepted?**

Yes, it is accepted but is more common in the rural village.

**Why?**

People are not well educated and civilized in the village like in the city. The city people don't usually marry many wives because they live like the Western people, although, if they want, they can do it. Nobody will question them. Every African girl knows that polygamy can happen in her marriage at any time.

**Did the multiple wives live in the same house?**

Yes, we all live together.

**What kind of struggles were there in day-to-day living arrangements with multiple wives and children?**

With the children, there are no struggles. They love playing and eating together. With the wives, we struggle with space and money. First, the house may not be large enough to occupy all of us. Secondly, the man may not give enough money. We struggled with space and money a lot.

**What did you do to get rid of or manage the struggles?**

There was nothing I could do as a woman. We just lived with it.

**Describe cultural traditions about marriage in some detail.**

When a woman finishes school from sixteen years upwards, men will be asking her out. They can go directly to her or go through her parents or from parents to parents. The parents of the man bring gifts to the parents of the girl. The man also gives gifts to the girl and takes her out. The parents fix the date for marriage, and the girl becomes a wife after the man pays her bride price, or dowry, and takes her home. If she has children, she will stay married to the man forever. If no children, she can be sent out or abandoned and replaced with another new wife. If all her children are girls, she and her girls will not inherit anything from the man when he dies.

**Can women remain unmarried into their twenties or thirties if she wishes to get advanced education and a career?**

Yes, and they go to the city to do that, not in the village. Nobody will marry them in the village.

**Would you ever count the children from other wives as part of your extended family on any level?**

No, it is against our belief.

**Why?**

I don't know why, but our people always say, "Don't count other people's children."

**If one of those other children called you now for help, do you believe you would help him or her?**

Yes, I will.

**How did your children feel about being part of that extended family with other wives and children when you were in Nigeria?**

I had only one girl. She liked that she has many siblings, but she didn't like that their father had many wives.

**Does your child ever talk about that part of her life now? How does she describe her feelings?**

When she talks about that part of her life now, she doesn't like it at all because she can now compare with here.

**Does your child feel any influence of Nigerian cultural traditions on her relationships in the U.S.?**

No.

**Do you feel any influence of Nigerian cultural traditions on your relationships with men in the U.S.?**

No.

**Would you provide encouragement to your daughter if she wishes to move back to Nigeria and have a traditional marriage?**

No, I will never.

**Could a wife in a traditional marriage in Nigeria with multiple wives ever refuse sex with her husband?**

No, never. She will be divorced, and no man will marry a divorced woman.

**What did wives of one husband typically fight about?**

They fight if the husband shows favoritism. They also fight about money if the husband gives more to one. Some fight when their children fight, but that doesn't last long.

**When you were slapped or caned by your husband, was there anyone you could ever go to for support?**

No, we don't go to anybody for support. What happens in the home stays in the home. That is one of the trainings we received as girls.

**Were there any laws that support a wife who was hurt by her husband? For example, could she ever call the police for support if severely beaten? In any of the large cities, were there any women's groups that support wives?**

No such laws at all. If we call police, they will not answer. If they answer, they will tell the woman to listen to her husband. No women's group that I knew of when I was home.

**Do you know if there is any current movement to change the cultural tradition of multiple wives?**

Yes, there are organizations talking about it and some new women groups.

**Please talk a little more about the use of traditional healers in villages versus Western medicine doctors. Do women typically use a traditional healer or Western medicine doctors for pregnancy and childbirth?**

Yes, they are powerful herbalists in the village. They claim to cure disease more than Western medicine. People say their medicines work. Pregnant women go to them for delivery because they cannot afford hospital. I used a prominent one in my village to deliver my child too. Their medicine doesn't work for HIV though. Anybody with HIV should go to the city hospital.

**What do you think are the benefits of going to a traditional healer versus Western medicine?**

The cost is cheaper, and the people are familiar with the herbs so they can trust the herbalists.

**Please discuss your faith traditions in Nigeria. For example, what do priests and pastors say about men having multiple wives?**

They preach against it in the city but not in the village. It is okay in the village because they too have multiple wives.

**Could a wife in Nigeria go to a priest or pastor for emotional support in dealing with a husband who has multiple wives and girlfriends?**

In the city, they can do that, but not in the village. What happens in the home stays in the home. In the village where it happens, the pastor would call them together and counsel them. That is all he can do. It is left for the couple to accept the counseling or not. The counseling is usually more about how the woman will be more obedient to the husband.

**Have you witnessed one?**

Yes, with my friend who lives in the city. She would always talk to their pastor about how her husband disrespects her in the presence of her junior wives. The pastor would call them together and advise my friend to be obedient to her husband so that he can stop disrespecting her.

**Could a woman in Nigeria choose college and career over marriage and be accepted?**

In the village, no woman can do that if she wants to have a husband. In the city, yes.

**Are girls in Nigeria encouraged to go onto vocational training or university?**

Yes, but mostly in the city. In the village, for the woman, it is more about settling down and having children.

# INTERVIEW NOTE

**Name**

P8

**What is your age?**

Thirty

**How long have you been in America?**

Four years

**What is your marital status?**

Married

**What is your present level of education?**

College

**What is your present occupation?**

LPN (Licensed practical nurse)

**How old were you when you got married in Nigeria?**

Twenty

**How old was your husband when you got married to him?**

Thirty-three

**Was that your first marriage? And how long?**

Yes. Six years.

**What was your education status?**

High school

**What was the education status of your husband?**

Teacher training school

**What was your occupation?**

School clerk

**What was the occupation of your husband?**

Teacher

**How many other wives did your husband have, and what were their ages?**

Three other wives. I don't know their ages.

**What was your position among the wives?**

I was the third wife.

**Who gave instructions among the wives?**

The most senior wife gave instruction among us. When she is not there, the second wife will do it. Instruction is in order of seniority.

**Can the most senior make decisions for the family?**

No, that is our husband's duty.

**Why?**

That is the culture.

**How many children lived in the home?**

Many children. I had none, but others had four children each.

**How would you describe your relationship with your husband in Nigeria?**

He was just there anytime I see him. He had no time for anybody. He was busy chasing his female students all about. He would come home shouting at everybody with fire in his eyes. He hated me because I didn't have a child. I didn't love him either. I just wanted to have children, but he died of HIV. Thank God he abandoned me before he got infected because I was tested and was HIV-negative.

**How would you describe the other wives of your husband in Nigeria?**

They were not good wives at all. They were cheating on my husband. I don't blame them because the man had no time for us. Immediately he left for work. The women would go too. Two of us were working. Others had shops outside, but they don't stay in the shops. They were busy satisfying themselves with other men. Now they all have HIV.

**Probe: Is it a common thing for women to have extramarital affairs?**

No, it is not acceptable for women at all. Women are supposed to be faithful. The man is the one who is allowed to have as many wives and girlfriends as he likes. Extramarital affairs by women is done secretly with young boys in the community, and if they are caught, they pay dearly for it.

**How do they pay dearly for it?**

They will be beaten in the presence of people in the community, and they will be divorced. It is a shameful thing on them and their parents. No man can ever marry them again because the husband will place a curse on them.

**Probe: Tell me about the curse. What is it like?**

It is just a statement made out of anger. If he says the woman will die young or become insane, so shall it be.

**Do you believe the curse?**

Yes, I believe it.

**Was the curse what kept you in your marriage, though you had no child with your husband and he was not faithful?**

Yes, the curse and childlessness.

**What happens to a childless woman?**

She is a nobody in the marriage.

**Probe: All women are nobody in their marriage anyway.**

True, but it is harder on a childless wife. The husband and his family will not treat her well, and if anything happens to any of the children in the house, she will be called the witch who let it happen. Other wives will also make fun of her childlessness. When the husband dies, the husband of the family will send her out with nothing. The only difference with her is she can remarry.

**Probe: So there is no curse on her as a witch?**

No, if she can have a child in her next marriage. If not, she will be labelled, and nobody will have anything to do with her anymore except for her family.

**Tell me about your relationship with other wives.**

I was fighting them because I know they were not faithful, and I didn't want to catch infection. They always assured me they were using protection. I kept their secret because, if I tell, they will turn it on me, and our husband will side with them and accuse me of jealousy. So somehow we pretended we were friends.

**Was the fight an ongoing thing?**

Yes.

**How did you do it? Physical or verbal?**

It was verbal. Nothing physical.

**How would you describe your experience of polygamy?**

It was really bad. I was very unhappy. Imagine not seeing your husband for days or seeing him in the midst of girls. Even when it was my turn for sex according to the roster, he will go out and come back very late and drunk. Then he removed me permanently from the roster because I couldn't bear him a child.

**Probe: Tell me about the roster.**

We all plan the roster together to know who will sleep with our husband on a particular day of the week. The husband also will agree to it. Our husband was so irresponsible that he will be too drunk to check the roster to know who was next. He will just pick any of us, and if the wife complains, he will beat her up and pick another wife.

**When he beats you up, do you go to hospital for treatment?**

No, I treat myself at home.

**Why? Don't you have the money to pay the bills? You were earning a living after all.**

Yes, but we don't go to hospital.

**Can you fight him legally for beating you up?**

No, we can't even talk to anyone about it. People will call us bad wives. There is a saying that what happens in the house stays in the house.

**When he beats you, do people come to your rescue?**

Yes, they come to our rescue but blame us the wife and tell us to listen to our husband.

**How did you cope living in polygamy?**

I hated it, but I was just praying and hoping that I would have a child.

**What was the role of your husband in polygamy?**

He was the head of the house and the master of all. Always treating us like his students. He is supposed to provide for all of us.

**Probe: Even when he allowed you to work?**

Yes, he is the head of the family, and according to our culture, he has to provide money for the family.

**Please tell me what you knew then about HIV/AIDS.**

We heard on the TV and radio that it is a killer disease transmitted by having sex with someone who is infected. Once you get it, you are dead. The villagers were running away from those who had it so the people started hiding their status and infecting other people. Even the hospitals were rejecting them. Men were advised to use condom, but they don't believe that they have infection, so they don't use condom, and no woman can ask them to use it. My brother committed suicide when he discovered that he had HIV. I am grateful to God that he was single. Other members of my family said he should have had a child after him. What for? To continue with the disease?

**Why did your brother commit suicide because of HIV?**

To avoid the shame. People will treat him like trash. They cannot get jobs or friends in the community.

**When people run away from them and hospitals reject them, what do they do?**

They turn to their family. Their family takes them to witch doctors for healing.

**Did you take your brother to a witch doctor?**

No. I don't believe in them.

**Did the witch doctors heal any HIV-infected person?**

No.

**What is your opinion about polygamy and HIV/AIDS?**

Polygamy is the reason there is so much AIDS in Nigeria. A man with many wives cannot satisfy the wives so the wives look for sex outside the marriage secretly and spread disease. The man too, because of his polygamous nature, continues to look for girls to marry all over the place and keep spreading disease.

**Probe: Can you fight your husband's girlfriends and tell them to leave your husband alone?**

No, I don't do that. My husband was to blame, not the girls.

**How did you perceive your risk for HIV/AIDS when you were in polygamy?**

I knew I was at risk, but that is what women are brought up for: satisfy your husband in bed, cook for him, have children for him, obey him, and expect his polygamous nature to marry many wives and give you STDs. You must not complain. I was at risk of HIV each time he had sex with me. Thank God he abandoned me at a time. That was the only reason I escaped HIV.

**How did your knowledge of HIV/AIDS affect your sexual relationship with your husband when you were in polygamy?**

I was afraid, but he never agreed to use condom. I was in constant fear of my husband losing it on me. One day he traveled out of the city and came back with tales of how he enjoyed himself with several girls. I felt hurt, but I couldn't talk so as not to send him back. At night, he said we should have sex. I refused him, and he started accusing me that I was seeing other men. If not, I should miss sex. I begged him that it was not because of that. I just wanted him to use condom since he has been with different girls. He beat me up so much and forced me to have sex. In the morning, he brought another woman into the house who became his wife eventually. For several months, he didn't touch me. Since then, I never brought up the idea of using condom. He became sick and died of AIDS. After his death, his family and my family wanted me to marry his brother, who was also a polygamist. I fled the country, and here I am, happily married. Thank God I didn't have a child for him. How could I have a child when he did not even have the time for me? Yet he blamed me for not having a child. Now I have a child with my present husband who treats me like an apple pie.

**Probe: Was there any prescription for protection from medical people or witch doctors?**

No. I don't go to them.

**Do you know any?**

Yes, I know some witch doctors who were popular in the village for their traditional healing powers. Many people, including my husband, go to them because they were cheaper than hospital, but they couldn't cure him.

**How is your relationship with your husband in your present marriage where you do not practice polygamy?**

He treats me like an apple pie, and I have a child with him. I'm pregnant with my second one.

# INTERVIEW NOTE

**Name**

P9

**What is your age?**

Thirty-four

**How long have you been in America?**

Three years

**What is your marital status?**

Married

**What is your present level of education?**

College

**What is your present occupation?**

LPN (Licensed practical nurse)

**How old were you when you got married?**

Twenty-one

**How old was your husband when you got married to him?**

Twenty-one

**Was that your first marriage? And how long?**

Yes. Ten years.

**What was your education status?**

High school

**What was the education status of your husband?**

High school

**What was your occupation?**

Trading

**What was the occupation of your husband?**

Motor spare parts trading

**How many other wives did your husband have, and what were their ages?**

Two other wives. I don't know their ages because we don't discuss it.

**What was your position among the wives?**

I was the first wife.

**As the first wife, were you the one giving instructions to the other wives?**

Yes.

**How many children lived in the home?**

We all had three children each.

**Where are your children now?**

They are all in Nigeria with my husband.

**Is he taking good care of them?**

Yes.

**How would you describe your relationship with your husband in Nigeria?**

It was not a good one. There were other wives competing with me. I could not talk to him alone without them listening through the wall. There was no love, no freedom, no voice. Nothing was good at all.

**How would you describe the other wives of your husband in Nigeria?**

The last wife was good at first. Later she joined the second wife against me because our husband called me a witch.

**Tell me about your relationship with other wives.**

Not good at all. Sometimes we fight, especially over the sex roster because our husband will just pick anyone to sleep with. Then it will turn to other things that we usually fight about, like sleeping outside.

**Probe: Tell me more about sleeping outside.**

When they don't get to sleep with him, they sleep outside.

**With whom?**

They have secret boyfriends outside that they thought I did not know. I see them when they go to their boys and give them gifts.

**Did you talk to them about it?**

No. If I talk, they will tell lies against me, and our husband will believe them.

**What will he do to you?**

He can send me out.

**Who would you go to if he sends you out?**

To my parents, but I will not allow that to happen because of my children. The children are the reason we women stay in our marriage.

**Probe: Tell me about the sex roster that you mentioned.**

That is the schedule for sleeping with our husband. Each one of us has a day to sleep with him, and we must keep to it, but he doesn't keep to it. He will just pick any of us, and we will have to make another one.

**Did you not involve him in the making of the roster?**

We tried, but he was not interested.

**How would you describe your experience of polygamy?**

Polygamy was a culture that women are trained to accept, whether we like it or not. I was one of the people who hated it because it is like treating a wife like a maid. My husband enjoyed it because it made him feel like a man. I cannot complain. I had to stick to rules in the house. Competition everywhere, and the husband cannot show love to any of the wives. Then there was fear of disease everywhere. Wives must be faithful, but husband cannot. It was a terrible experience for me.

**Did you talk to him about your experience?**

No, I can't talk to him because, for him, he was doing the normal thing a polygamous man does.

**Was your experience the reason you left him?**

I won the visa lottery and came here.

**When you told him about the visa lottery, how did he react?**

He was happy for me.

**Was it in your plan to bring him here too?**

No.

**Did you tell him that?**

No, he will not allow me to come if I tell him that.

**Probe: So you saw the visa lottery as a way of escape.**

Yes. I was very unhappy in the marriage.

**How did you cope living in polygamy?**

I lived with it, hoping nothing bad happened.

**What was the role of your husband in polygamy?**

He was the headmaster of the house. He was responsible for feeding us and providing the money.

**Was he providing the money?**

Yes.

**How did he give money that all of you spent?**

He was giving me the first wife money for food on Mondays. I will then take the other wives with me to the market to buy the food.

**What about money for personal upkeep?**

We were all traders, and he allowed us so we had our own money. Sometimes he would get money from me, which he never pays back.

**If you ask for your money, will he not pay you back?**

No. It is enough that he allowed me to work.

**Please tell me what you knew then about HIV/AIDS.**

It is a killer disease.

**Probe: How did you know?**

Through the TV and radio. We heard, if you have sex with a carrier, you will get infected and die soon. People were treating the carriers like outcasts, so they started hiding it. But if you keep to one wife, you will not get it. The problem is the culture does not allow that. The people were falling sick and dying, yet men were marrying wives and boasting. The wives are infected, including the children, and a whole family was being wiped out by this terrible disease, right under our nose. Some of us started fighting the prostitutes, and it actually worked.

**How were the people treating the carriers like outcasts?**

They were not giving HIV-infected people jobs and housing. Not even sitting with them. Their families are the ones who take care of them to the point of paying traditional healers for them.

**Were the traditional healers healing them?**

No.

**How did you fight the prostitutes?**

We would go to them secretly with area young boys and beat them up.

**Did your husband know about it?**

No. If he knows about it, we are in trouble.

**What would he do?**

He can beat us up too.

**When he beats you up, do you go to hospital?**

If I am injured, I would go to hospital.

**Who pays the bill?**

I do.

**What about him? Can't he pay?**

No, it is enough that he didn't send me out.

**Probe: Can you report him or take any legal action against him if he beats you up?**

No, there is no court for that. We don't even talk about it because the society frowns at any woman who talks about her husband. What happens in the house stays in the house.

**What is your opinion about polygamy and HIV/AIDS?**

Polygamy is the cause of HIV/AIDS. If the man is rich, the wives are in trouble because there are girls out there who want to enjoy the money as well. How can one man satisfy all those girls and wives so the women also look for sex outside? We don't know who is infecting who. Everybody is spreading the disease and keeping it to themselves until they fall sick, and everybody knows because the hospitals reject them. Then they will go to traditional healers.

**Are traditional healers the witch doctors?**

Yes.

**Do you believe that their medicine works?**

I don't know. I have never used their medicine, but the people claim it works. My husband claims it works too.

**Was he using it?**

I think so, but I am not sure.

**How did you perceive your risk for HIV/AIDS when you were in polygamy?**

I knew I was at risk and my husband was at risk too, but he will not admit it because of his ego. We women already know that our husbands will bring another wife as soon as possible, so we are prepared for it. Polygamy can never be done away with. It is like killing the men's ego. They will look for another way of doing it. Men are polygamous by nature because they do not get pregnant and the society does not frown against their promiscuity. In some parts of Nigeria, it is the joy of the parents when their son has numerous wives. It shows that he is a real man. Do you know that parents even boast of it? So knowing all these, I know I was in a risky marriage where I can get HIV easily, but as a woman, I dare not ask for protection if I don't want trouble.

**What kind of trouble?**

If I ask him to use condom, he will suspect me of extramarital affairs and divorce me.

**Can you remarry if he divorces you?**

No. Men don't like to marry divorced women.

**How did your knowledge of HIV/AIDS affect your sexual relationship with your husband when you were in polygamy?**

I was afraid, but it did not affect sex because I had to have children. I can't let him divorce me because the society will not accept me as a single woman. Even if I stop having children, I don't know how we would have done it. The decision would be his. It's either he would abandon me or he will be using something so that I won't get pregnant.

**Probe: So you did not protect yourself, knowing that he could have HIV/AIDS?**

No, if I do that and he gets to know, he will suspect me of cheating. I suspected that he was using a traditional healer protection because he always boasted that he can't have HIV, but as for me, I did not do anything of such.

**How is your relationship with your husband in your present marriage where you do not practice polygamy?**

We love each other, and there is freedom. I can have my husband to myself.

# INTERVIEW NOTE

**Name**

P10

**What is your age?**

Forty-five

**How long have you been in America?**

Four years

**What is your marital status?**

Married

**What is your present level of education?**

High school

**What is your present occupation?**

Fashion business

**How old were you when you got married?**

Twenty

**How old was your husband when you got married to him?**

Forty

**Was this your first marriage? And how long?**

Yes. Twenty-one years.

**What was your education status?**

Teacher training

**What was the education status of your husband?**

High school

**What was your occupation?**

Teacher

**What was the occupation of your husband?**

Business

**How many other wives did your husband have, and what were their ages?**

Two other wives. The first one was older, and the last one was younger than me.

**What was your position among the wives?**

The second wife

**Who was giving instructions among the wives?**

The first wife gave instructions about cleaning and cooking and taking care of our husband.

**Was there a favorite wife among you?**

I was the favorite before the last wife came and took over. Though our husband did not show favoritism, we usually have the feeling.

**How many children lived in the home?**

My children were six. We don't count children for their mothers in our culture.

**Where are your children now?**

Three in U.S. One in Canada; the rest in Nigeria.

**How would you describe your relationship with your husband in Nigeria?**

It was not bad. He was a nice man. He was taking care of me and other wives.

**How would you describe the other wives of your husband in Nigeria?**

I was the second wife. The first one was like a mother to all of us. She is a very nice woman. The third wife was nice and respectful, but she always stays with our husband even when we needed him. She is the last wife so she is the favorite. Our husband did not show favoritism anyway. When she first came, she was lousy and behaving like a prostitute, but as she grew, she got matured.

**Tell me about your relationship with other wives.**

Good. There was no fight. Little jealousies here and there, but nothing big. The last wife usually starts something like getting close to me or the other wife when she wants to gossip. You know when you are three in a place, one of you will want to be the middleman.

**Did you allow her?**

No, we both make fun of her.

**How did your husband react to that?**

He did not know about it.

**How would you describe your experience of polygamy?**

My experience was not bad because my husband played it well. He treated us equally and took care of us, but if not for the culture, I will not do it. I want somebody I can call my own and not our own. There was no intimacy. We were not fighting because we feared and respected our husband. He was one of the best rich men around, and no woman will want to lose such a man. I was clean, my husband was clean, but I cannot trust other wives. If they were having boyfriends when our husband was getting old, that was a problem for us.

**How was it a problem?**

Because they will bring disease.

**How did you cope living in polygamy?**

We had a roster like a meal plan for sex, and we kept to it. Our children loved one another. I was always praying and watching other wives because I did not want anyone to bring disease for me.

**Did you suspect or catch any of them being unfaithful?**

I did not catch any of them, and I think the first wife was clean and decent, but the last wife was young and beautiful, so there is the possibility that she is unfaithful.

**What made you think she could be unfaithful?**

Our husband was getting old when he married her, and it was possible he could not satisfy her sexually, but that was just my suspicion.

**What was the role of your husband in polygamy?**

He was our breadwinner, and he provided for all of us.

**And he allowed you to work?**

Yes. The first wife and I worked. The last wife was the only housewife.

**Please tell me what you knew then about HIV/AIDS.**

They said it is a killer disease

**Probe: Who said?**

TV, radio, all these people who work in the hospital. Many people were dying of it. Once you have sex with a prostitute, you catch it, and as a man with many wives, you get home and spread it to your wives. Everybody runs away from them, even the hospital people.

**Everybody runs away from whom?**

People with HIV.

**How do they earn a living if people run away from them?**

Nobody gives them a job. No hospital treats them except traditional healers. Their family members are the ones who take care of them. My sister who had three children contracted HIV from her husband but did not disclose it until she came down with illnesses.

**How did you know that your sister contracted HIV from her husband?**

My sister's husband was promiscuous. He had a friend who was a witch doctor, and people were telling rumors that the witch doctor was giving him traditional medicine to cure AIDS.

**Do you believe traditional medicine cured HIV?**

No. My sister died despite all that we spent on traditional medicine.

**Who took care of your sister?**

When her husband and other wives abandoned her, I took her in with her children and cared for them all until she died. I left the children in my mother's care when I relocated here.

**What is your opinion about polygamy and HIV/AIDS?**

Polygamy is what helps HIV/AIDS to spread like wildfire. If people keep to their wives and husband, there will be no problem, but if one of them goes outside to have sex, then everybody will be infected and die.

**How did you perceive your risk for HIV/AIDS when you were in polygamy?**

Polygamy is the system that we are used to, so women know the risk. We don't have the right to complain as women if we don't want to be sent out. I was not at risk as long as my husband and co-wives were keeping to themselves, but can you trust other wives? Younger wives usually have sex with older children of their husbands if their husbands are too old to sexually satisfy them. They look for the one who looks very much like the husband so that, if they get pregnant by accident, the child will look like their husband, and there will be no suspicion. What if the boy has a girlfriend who is a prostitute and has HIV? Then the wife will catch it and give it to our husband and then all of us. I don't know if that happened with the third wife. She was very young when he married her, and he was fifty-six then.

**With your perception of risk, why did you stay in the marriage?**

My husband was very rich and was taking care of me, and I had children with him.

**How did your knowledge of HIV/AIDS affect your sexual relationship with your husband when you were in polygamy?**

We did not use protection at all, though I feared HIV. I could not bring it up with my husband because he would think I was doubting him. I was just being the obedient wife and was following our plan in the house for sex. At the early stage of my marriage, I did not fear much until the third wife arrived. From the moment I saw her, I knew we were doomed. She was always talking and behaving like a prostitute. I don't know why my gentle husband married such a lousy slut. How we all escaped HIV/AIDS, I don't know 'til today, but I was always praying anytime my husband had sex with me. I thank God that He answered my prayers. My husband was very rich and was taking care of all of us. I always feel that he would not have been a polygamist if not for the culture. Anyway, my present husband is the best. I am free of fear, and I can talk. Thank God for America.

**You talked about a plan for sex. Tell me more.**

It is a roster that we make with our husband for who sleeps with him when.

**If he thinks you were doubting him, what will he do to you?**

He will be unhappy with me. I don't know what he can do, but that will affect our relationship.

**Why did you leave him?**

I won the visa lottery and came here. I left two of my children with him because I was sure he would take care of them. My first child had married before I left, and one of my children was already in Canada with family. Two of them came here with me, and another one joined them here recently.

# REFERENCES

Aderemi, T. J., and B. J. Pillay. "Sexual Abstinence and HIV Knowledge In School-Going Adolescents with Intellectual Disabilities and Non-Disabled Adolescents in Nigeria." *Journal of Child & Adolescent Mental Health* 25(2) (2013): 161–174. doi:10.2989/17280583.2013.823867.

AIDS.gov. "What is HIV/AIDS?" http://aids.gov/hiv-aids-basics/hiv -aids-101/what-is-hiv-aids.

AIDS Healthcare Foundation. "Nigeria." http://www.aidshealth.org /africa/Nigeria.

Akoto, A. "Why Don't They Change? Law Reform, Tradition and Widows Rights in Ghana. *Feminist Legal Studies* 21(3)(2013): 263–264. doi:10.1007/s10691-013-9252-y.

Anyanwu, J. C. "Marital Status, Household Size, and Poverty in Nigeria: Evidence from the 2009/2010 Survey Data Working Paper Series N° 180." Tunis, Tunisia: African Development Bank, 2013.

Attah, N. "Contesting Exclusion in a Multi-ethnic State: Rethinking Ethnic Nationalism in Nigeria." *Social Identities* 19(5)(2013): 607–620. doi:10.1080/13504630.2013.835515.

Audu, B. M., A. U. El-Nafaty, B. G. Bako, G. S. Melah, A. G. Mairiga, and A. A. Kullima. "Attitude of Nigerian women to Contraceptive Use by men." *Journal of Obstetrics*

& *Gynaecology, 28*(6)(2008): 621–625. doi:10.1080/01443610802283530.

AVERT. "HIV and AIDS in Nigeria." http://www.avert.org/aids-nigeria.htm.

Awusi, V. O., and E. B. Anyanwu. "HIV/AIDS-related Knowledge and Attitudes of Pregnant Women in Delta State, Nigeria." *Benin Journal of Postgraduate Medicine* 11(1)(2009), Art. No. 3. http://dx.doi.org/10.4314/bjpm.v11i1.48821.

Bazeley, P., and K. Jackson. *Qualitative data analysis with NVivo*, 2nd ed. London: Sage, 2013.

Bentz, V. M., and J. J. Shapiro. *Mindful Enquiry in Social Research*. Thousand Oaks, Calif.: Sage, 1998.

Berry, N., A. Jenkins, J. Martin, C. Davis, D. Wood, G. Schild, and N. Almond. "Mitochondrial DNA and Retroviral RNA Analyses of Archival Oral Polio Vaccine (OPV CHAT) Materials: Evidence of Macaque Nuclear Sequences Confirms Substrate Identity." *Vaccine* 23 (2005): 1639–1648. http://dx.doi.org10.1016/j.vaccine.2004.10.038.

Bowen, E. A. "AIDS at 30: Implications for Social Work Education." *Journal of Social Work Education* 49(2013): 265–276. http://dx.doi.org/10.1080/10437797.2013.768116.

Cao, Z., Y. Chen, and S. Wang. "Health Belief Model Based Evaluation of School Health Education Programme for Injury Prevention among High School Students in the Community Context." *BMC Public Health, 14*(1)(2014): 1–15. doi:10.1186/1471-2458-14-26.

Centers for Disease Control and Prevention. "Basic Information about HIV and AIDS." http://www.cdc.gov/hiv/topics/basic/index.htm

Chavan, L. B. "History of HIV and AIDS." *National Journal of Community Medicine* 2(2011): 502–503. http://www.njcmindia.org

Creswell, J. *Research Design: Qualitative, Quantitative, and Mixed Methods Approaches*, 3rd ed. Thousand Oaks, Calif.: Sage, 2009.

Creswell, J. W. *Qualitative Inquiry and Research Design: Choosing among Five Approaches*, 3rd ed. Thousand Oaks, Calif.: Sage, 2013.

D'Angelo, P., J. C. Pollock, K. Kiernicki, and D. Shaw. "Framing of AIDS in Africa." *Politics and the Life Sciences* 32(1) (2014): 100–125. http://dx.doi.org/10.2990/32_2_100.

De Cock, K. M., H. W. Jaffe, and J. W. Curran. "Reflections on 30 Years of AIDS." *Emerging Infectious Diseases* 17(2011): 1044–1048. http://dx.doi.org/10.3201 /eid1706.100184.

Do, M., and D. Meekers. "Multiple Sex Partners and Perceived Risk of HIV Infection in Zambia: Attitudinal Determinants and Gender Differences." *AIDS Care* 21(10)(2009).

Doosuur, A., and A. S. Arome. "Curbing the Cultural Practices of Wife Inheritance and Polygamy Through Information Dissemination in Benue State." *IOSR Journal of Humanities and Social Science* 13(1)(2013): 50–54. http://dx.doi.org/10.9790/0837-1315054.

Doyle, S. "Member Checking with Older Women: A Framework for Negotiating Meaning." *Health Care for Women International* 8(10)(2007): 888–908.

Federal Republic of Nigeria. "Global AIDS response Country Progress Report (GARPR, 2012)." http://www.unaids.org/en/dataanalysis.

Giorgi, A. P. and B. M. Giorgi. "The Descriptive Phenomenological Psychological Method," in *Qualitative Research in Psychology: Expanding Perspectives in Methodology and Design*, ed. P.M. Camic, J.E. Rhodes, and L. Yardley. Washington, DC: American Psychological Association, 2003.

Green, M. "Religion, Family Law, and Recognition of Identity in Nigeria." *Emory International Law Review* 25(2)(2011): 945–966.

Hajizadeh, M., D. Sia, S. J. Heymann, and A. Nandi. "Socioeconomic inequalities in HIV/AIDS Prevalence in sub-Saharan African Countries: Evidence from the Demographic Health Surveys." *International Journal for Equity in Health* 13*(2014),* 18–40. http://dx.doi.org/10.1186/1475-9276-13-18.

Hayden, J. A. *Introduction to Health Behavior Theory*, 2nd ed. Burlington, Mass.: Jones & Bartlett Learning, 2014.

Hoyt, A., and S. M. Patterson. "Mormon Masculinity: Changing Gender Expectations in the Era of Transition from Polygamy to Monogamy, 1890–1920." *Gender & History* 23(1)(2011): 72–91.

Hycner, R.H. "Some Guidelines for the Phenomenological Analysis of Interview Data." *Human Studies* 8(3)(1985): 279–303.

Ilevbare, M. "Practice of Polygamy in Nigeria." http://www.lifepaths360.com/index.php/practice-of-polygamy-in-nigeria-10510.

Jegede, A. S. "Problems and Prospects of Healthcare Delivery in Nigeria: Issues in Political Economy and Social Inequality," in *Currents and Perspectives in Sociology*, ed. U.C. Isiugho-Abanihe, A. N. Isamah, J. O. Adesina, 212–226. Ikeja: Malthouse Press Ltd., 2002.

Kanki, P. J. "HIV/AIDS Global Epidemic," in *Infectious Diseases: Selected Entries from the Encyclopedia of Sustainability Science and Technology*, ed. P. Kanki and D. J. Grimes, 27–62. New York: Springer, 2013.

Katrak, S. M. "The Origin of HIV and AIDS: An Enigma of Evolution." *Annals of Indian Academy of Neurology* 9(2006): 5–10. http://www.annalsofian.org.

Knight, L. *UNAIDS: The First 10 years, 1996–2006*. Geneva, Switzerland: UNAIDS, 2008.

Lawani, L. O., A. K. Onyebuchi, and C. A. Iyoke. (2014). "Dual Method Use for Protection of Pregnancy and Disease Prevention among HIV-Infected Women in South East Nigeria. *BMC Women's Health* 14(2014), Art. No. 39. http://dx.doi.org/10.1186/1472-6874-14-39.

Mairig, A. G., A. A. Kullima, B. Bako, and M. A. Kolo. "Sociocultural Factors Influencing Decision-Making Related to Fertility among the Kanuri Tribe of North-Eastern Nigeria." *African Journal of Primary Health Care & Family Medicine* 2(1)(2010), Art. No. 94. http://dx.doi.org/10.4102/phcfm.v2i1.94.

Miles, M. B., and A. M. Huberman. *Qualitative Data Analysis: An Expanded Sourcebook*. Thousand Oaks, Calif.: Sage, 1994.

Moustakas, C. *Phenomenological Research Methods*. Thousand Oaks, Calif.: Sage, 1994.

Namisi, F. S., A. J. Flisher, S. Overland, S. Bastien, and H. Onya. "Sociodemographic Variations in Communication on Sexuality and HIV/AIDS with Parents, Family Members And Teachers among In-School Adolescents:

A Multi-site Study in Tanzania and South Africa. *Scand J Public Health* 37 (2009), 265–74.

Nkhoma, K., J. Seymour, and A. Arthur. "An Educational Intervention to Reduce Pain and Improve Pain Management for Malawian People Living with HIV/AIDS and Their Family Carers: Study Protocol for a Randomized Controlled Trial. *Trials* 14(2013): 216–223. http://dx.doi.org/10.1186/1745-6215-14-216.

Nuttall, P., A. Shankar, and M. B. Beverland. Mapping the Unarticulated Potential of Qualitative Research. *Journal of Advertising Research* 51(2011): 153–163.

Nyathikazi, T. J. L. "Investigating the Association between HIV and AIDS and Polygamy among Practising Polygamists in Kwazulu-Natal, North Coast Area," Master's thesis, Stellenbosch University, Stellenbosch, South Africa, 2013, http://ir1.sun.ac.za/handle/10019.1/80190

Obidoa, C. A., and R. G. Cromley. A Geographical Analysis of HIV/AIDS Infection in Nigeria, 1991–2001." *Journal of Social, Behavioral & Health Sciences* 6(2012), 13–29. http://dx.doi.org/10.5590/JSBHS.2012.06.1.02.

Obire, O., U. Nwakwo, J. Ramesh, and R. Putbeti. "Incidence of HIV and AIDS in Ahoada, Port Harcourt, Nigeria." *Electronic Journal of Biology (eJBio)* 5(2)(2009): 28–33.

Odimegwu, C., S. A. Adedini, and D. N. Ononokpono. HIV/AIDS Stigma and Utilization of Voluntary Counselling and Testing in Nigeria. *BMC Public Health* 13(2013): 465–479. http://dx.doi.org/10.1186/1471-2458-13-465.

Ostrach, B., and M. Singer. "At Special Risk: Biopolitical Vulnerability and HIV/STI Syndemics among Women." *Health Sociology Review* 21(3)(2012): 258–271.

Patton, M. Q. *Qualitative Research and Evaluation Methods*, 3rd ed. Thousand Oaks, Calif.: Sage, 2002.

Parker, R. G., D. Easton, and C. H. Klein. "Structural Barriers and Facilitators in HIV Prevention: A Review of International Research." *Official Journal of the International AIDS Society* 14(1)(2000): S22–S32.

Pennington, J. "HIV & AIDS in Nigeria." Avert HIV/AIDS International. www.avert.org/aidsnigeria.htm.

Reynolds, P. D. *A Primer in Theory Construction*. Boston: Pearson, 2007.

Rosenstock, I. "Historical Origins of the Health Belief Model." *Health Education Monographs* 2(1974): 328–335.

Rudestam, K., and R. Newton. *Surviving Your Dissertation: A Comprehensive Guide to Content and Process*, 3rd ed. Los Angeles: Sage, 2007.

Saddiq A., R. Tolhurst, D. Lalloo, and S. Theobald. "Promoting Vulnerability or Resilience to HIV? A Qualitative study on Polygamy in Maiduguri, Nigeria." *AIDS Care* 2(2010): 146–151. http://dx.doi.org/10.1080/09540120903039844.

Sharma, M. "Health Belief Model: Need for More Utilization in Alcohol and Drug Education. *Journal of Alcohol and Drug Education* 55(1)(2011): 3–6.

Siegle, D. "Qualitative versus Quantitative." Gifted Education, University of Connecticut. www.gifted.uconn.edu.

Smith, J., K. Ahmed, and A. Whiteside. "Why HIV/AIDS Should Be Treated as Exceptional: Arguments from sub-Saharan Africa and Eastern Europe. *African Journal of AIDS Research* 10(2011): 345–356. http://dx.doi.org/10.2989/16085906.2011.637736.

Strauss, G. "Is Polygamy Inherently Unequal?" *Ethics* 122(2012): 516–544. http://dx.doi.org/10.1086/664754.

Ugwoke, B. U. "Reducing the Effects of HIV/AIDS in Nigeria: The Role of Libraries and Information Centres." *International Journal of Information Management* 34(2014): 308–310. doi:10.1016/j.ijinfomgt.2013.09.005.

US Census Bureau. "Urban and rural classification." https://www.census.gov/geo/reference/urban-rural.html.

US Department of Health and Human Services (DHHS). "HIV/AIDS Basics." http://aids.gov/hiv-aids-basics/hiv-aids-101/what-is-hiv-aids.

UNAIDS. "Global Report: Regional HIV & AIDS Statistics 2001 and 2009." http://www.unaids.org

———. "Global Report: UNAIDS Report on the Global AIDS Epidemic 2013. http://www.unaids.org

Winn, Jr., W., S. Allen, W. Janda, E. Koneman, G. Procop, P. Schreckenberger, and G. Woods. *Koneman's Color Atlas and Textbook of Diagnostic Microbiology*, 6th ed. Philadelphia: Lippincott Williams & Wilkins, 2006.

Wolfe, N. D., W. M. Switzer, J. K. Carr, V. B. Bhullar, V. Shanmugam, U. Tamoufe, and W. Heneine. "Naturally Acquired Simian Retrovirus Infections in Central African Hunters." *Lancet* 363(2004): 932–937. http://dx.doi.org/10.1016/S0140-6736(04)15787-5.